Secrets of the Beauty Insiders

Simple and Straightforward Top to Toe Tips for the Rest of Us

Nada Guirgis Manley

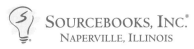
SOURCEBOOKS, INC.
NAPERVILLE, ILLINOIS

Published by Sourcebooks, Inc.
P.O. Box 4410, Naperville, Illinois 60567-4410
(630) 961-3900
Fax: (630) 961-2168
www.sourcebooks.com

Library of Congress Cataloging-in-Publication Data

Manley, Nada.
  Secrets of the beauty insiders : simple and straightforward top to toe tips
for the rest of us / Nada Manley.
     p. cm.
  ISBN-13: 978-1-4022-0781-5
  ISBN-10: 1-4022-0781-6
  1. Beauty, Personal. 2. Skin--Care and hygiene. I. Title.

RA776.98.M36 2006
646.7'26--dc22

2006021020

Printed and bound in the United States of America.
D.B.H. 10 9 8 7 6 5 4 3 2 1

Dedication

To my husband, Kevin, for his unwavering support, encouragement, and, when I needed it, the occasional push; to my parents, Dr. Wagid Guirgis and Suzan Guirgis, my earliest fans; to Nash, for giving me the experience that made this book possible, and for a friendship I will always cherish; to my sister, Nelly, and my cousins, Lois, Nancy, and Anne, for friendship, laughter, and, most of all, for tolerating years of unsolicited beauty advice and know-it-all-ness; to my brother, Dr. Faheem Guirgis, for looking over some of the technical stuff in this book, and for always making me proud; to my baby, Lola Suzan, who, before she was even born, inspired and motivated me through the process of getting this book published; to my agent, June Clark, for being the first to believe in this project; and finally, to God, for a life filled with love and blessings.

Acknowledgments

This book, more than most, was really a collaborative process, so I have many people to thank. First of all, I'd like to acknowledge my agent, June Clark at the Peter Rubie Literary Agency, for her vision, guidance, and support, and my editor, Bethany Brown, for a sharp eye and plenty of patience. I'd also like to thank the dozens of kind, talented, generous people who make up the Beauty Bunch, with a special nod to Hara Glick, for helping me get the ball rolling; June Jacobs, Jan Marini, and Peter Thomas Roth, the first experts on board; Shan Albert, for freely sharing her knowledge of natural skin-care ingredients and answering countless questions; Diane Ranger and Hollis Wright, for the most thorough coverage of color theory and mineral makeup that I have ever seen; Dee Pearn, for her dedication to accuracy and her professionalism; Bobbe Joy and Barry Reitman, for making me feel welcome in L.A. and giving me the star treatment; Ouidad, for giving me "shampoo-commercial" hair and showing my readers how to do the same; Dr. Jeffrey Dover, for saving my skin before my wedding and then contributing his wisdom to my book; Rebecca James Gadberry, for helping me make sense of product labels; Kari Boatner, for her commitment to her art, and for her friendship; Giella, for her kindness and her genius; Debra Macki, for some of the best, most thorough makeup information I have ever seen; Angela Nice, for her fabulous insight into cellulite; Gabrielle Ophals, for her kindness and her knowledge; Meg Thompson, for great tips and for answering dozens of emails; Charles Worthington, for drinks at the Whiskey in Chicago and contributing his eye-opening survey; and Jimmy Vanegas, for sharing his impressive list of clients and friends, many of whom appear in this book. And finally, I'd like to thank all the P.R. pros who arranged dozens of interviews, answered hundreds of emails, and pretty much made this whole book possible, especially the teams at Kip Morrison, Behrman, Tractenberg, Blue Sky, Carolyn Kamii, Carolyn Leber, Kodora, Morehouse, Kaplow, CMM, M. Craig, J9, Siren, Lola Red, and finally, Jennifer Mayer and Michelle Bondarchuk at Frédéric Fekkai.

Table of Contents

Introduction

The Trials of a Beauty Editor

At the age of ten, I received my first makeup kit: a purse-sized collection of bronze shades from Coty. It was to play with, of course, not to wear, but I felt glamorous and grown-up. At twenty, I was giving unsolicited beauty advice to my sorority sisters with the certainty that can only come from youth and inexperience. At twenty-two, I was a beauty editor. I spent my days doing what I'd always done, reading up on the latest beauty trends, collecting beauty tips, and playing with makeup. But now it was not simply a means of blowing off homework. It was my job. When the first big box of beauty booty arrived, I dived in with the abandon of a true addict.

That was more than a dozen years ago. Since then, I've rubbed and scrubbed, tried and tested my way through thousands of products. I have interviewed hundreds of beauty experts and endured countless treatments. I've been a human guinea pig, submitting my face, my hair, and my body to endless poking, prodding, rubbing, and tugging, all for the cause of beauty. Along the way, I've discovered duds and dream products, failures and finds. All of this trial and error has made me one picky beauty fanatic. As tempting as a "revolutionary" new skin treatment may seem, I need more than miraculous claims to be sold. I need evidence. So I read the fine print and speak to the experts. Most important, I try it for myself, because a treatment is only fabulous if it works.

Through it all, I've retained my fascination with beauty. My heart still leaps when I hear about the latest miracle skin-saving ingredient or learn that a certain admired celeb attributes her glow to a particular shade of blush. I've remained a beauty consumer first, an editor second.

Secrets of the Beauty Insiders is written for consumers. Although simple and straightforward, it's not for everyone.

There's a small percentage of women who have mastered their makeup and skin-care routines. Their look is beautiful, flattering, and suits their lifestyle. They are open to change without being a slave to trends. They have developed an effective skin-care program, which they adjust seasonally. They skim fashion magazines for information on advances in skin care and the latest makeup looks, and pick and choose only what works for them.

I don't know any of these women.

Secrets of the Beauty Insiders is for the rest of us. If you fall, even loosely, into one of the following categories, this book is for you.

for a jog, run for office, organize your spice rack. If you think that beauty is a superficial, frivolous waste of time, then you haven't met your perfect moisturizer. Every fresh-scrubbed beauty needs a good skin-care routine. And a little makeup, artfully applied, can look natural and polished. Even if you don't know an eye cream from a pimple cream, and you're too afraid to ask, this book will help you tap into your inner glamour girl.

IF LOVING BEAUTY IS WRONG, I DON'T WANNA BE RIGHT.

You are a beauty "junkie." Constantly on the search for the next big thing, you're always experimenting with new products and new looks. Sometimes, your experiments are successful, like that dusty tube of moisturizer you discovered in a health-food store that's become a staple, or the blush you snagged from your best friend that gives you that perfect, just-went-for-a-run flush. Other times, as in the unfortunate orange lipstick incident, the results of your experimentation are less than impressive. This book will encourage that spirit of creativity while helping you zero in on potential pitfalls.

BUT I'VE ALWAYS WORN IT THIS WAY!

You know what you want and what looks good on you. You discovered your favorite shade of lipstick at twenty-five when you were on your honeymoon and your new husband paid you a compliment. Unfortunately, the honeymoon is over. Ten years have passed, maybe twenty, and you're still sporting the same look. You know a good thing when you see it, so it should be easy to choose some new looks from the choices on the following pages. Modern makeup colors and formulas can freshen your look, update your attitude, and maybe even send you packing for a second honeymoon.

WHO ME, MAKEUP?

You're a soap-and-water girl. A beauty holdout. After all, who needs makeup when you're naturally beautiful? While other girls spend hours in front of the mirror, you stick your hair in a ponytail and go

THE SECRETS BREAKDOWN

Don't worry. Whether your issue is excess or neglect, or whether you're simply curious if there's something better out there, *Secrets of the Beauty Insiders* can help.

Here's how it works. Each of the eleven chapters focuses on a single category (skin care, hair care, eye makeup, etc.). Within each chapter, you'll find three elements:

1. **Insider Information from the Beauty Bunch:** insider advice and top tips from an elite group of over seventy-five beauty-industry experts. These pros represent the best of the industry, and range from skin-care stars to makeup mavens to product pioneers. They spill their secrets, offering priceless tips and detailed techniques. You'll find household names like Oribe, Peter Thomas Roth, and Wende Zomnir sharing space with industry insiders like Julie Hewett, Diane Ranger, and Debra Luftman. [See "The Beauty Bunch" on this page for a comprehensive list of the experts featured in *Secrets of the Beauty Insiders*.]

2. **The Buzz from the Beauty Editor:** my personal commentary on dozens of beauty issues, from disastrous cuts to magnificent manicures. You'll get tips, techniques, and opinions based on my years of experience as a beauty editor, and a few product recommendations as well.

3. **What the Pros Choose:** product picks from the Beauty Bunch in fifty-five categories.

Secrets of the Beauty Insiders is a reference book, a resource, and a compilation of tips——the choice is yours. Use it as you see fit.

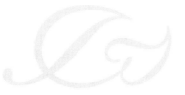

THE BEAUTY BUNCH

- **Shan Albert:** the director of education and product development for Zed Laboratories, the world's leader in revolutionary advances in skin care. She has over a quarter century of experience in esthetics and as a licensed esthetician, salon owner, educator, and product developer. Albert is also an international speaker on esthetics and ingredient and product knowledge.

- **Kathryn Alice:** beauty publicist, the Alice Company.

- **Terri Apanasewicz:** celebrity makeup artist with L.A.'s Cloutier Agency, Apanasewicz has appeared in *InStyle*, *Forbes*, and on HGTV. She was also featured in stylist Phillip Bloch's book, *Elements of Style*. Her famous clients have included Michael Michele, Jeri Ryan, Kristin Davis, Toni Braxton, and Reba McEntire.

- **Nick Arrojo:** British-born hair guru and owner of the Arrojo Studio in New York City whose clients include actress Minnie Driver and *Sports Illustrated* supermodel Melissa Keller. Arrojo is also the hair expert on TLC's popular *What Not to Wear*.

- **Clarissa Azar:** one of the founders of Fake Bake, a premier line of self-tanning products favored by Britney Spears and Madonna. Fake Bake has been featured in the *New York Times*, *Lucky*, *Vogue*, and *Harper's Bazaar*, as well as on *The View*.

- **Jeanie Barnett:** director of corporate communications, Tweezerman.

- **Marsha Bialo:** Hollywood-based celebrity manicurist affiliated with OPI whose work has graced the hands of Kate Hudson, Beyonce, Renee Zellweger, Jessica Simpson, Gretchen Mol, Gwen Stefani, Eva Longoria, Teri Hatcher, and Alicia Keys. Her artistry has appeared on the pages of *Vogue*, *Glamour*, *Town & Country*, *Cosmopolitan*, *Elle*, *Self*, and *Nylon*, and in ad campaigns for Ralph Lauren and Giorgio Armani. She was awarded Best Nail Design by *Los Angeles Magazine* in 2003.

- **Darin Birchler:** star hairstylist from the Chop Chop Salon Gallery in Los Angeles who was named L.A.'s Hot New Up-and-Comer by *Los Angeles Magazine*.

- **Kari Boatner:** permanent-cosmetics pioneer who has developed innovative instruments and artistic procedures for the application of permanent make-up. Boatner is board certified by the American Academy of Micropigmentation, and is one of only sixty board-certified micropigmentation instructors in the nation. She has been featured in *Elle* as one of the country's top permanent-cosmetic technicians.

- **Spresa Bojkovic:** hair colorist and salon owner known for her trademark natural color. Bojkovic has worked in the hair-care industry since the age of fourteen. Her career took her from a local Staten Island salon, Gigi, to the prestigious Robert Kree Salon in New York City. At twenty-three, Bojkovic opened the Damian West Salon, combining the warm atmosphere of Gigi with the glamour of Robert Kree.

- **Danielle Browning:** spa director of Boston's famed G Spa. Browning has been featured in *Allure*, *Elle*, *Boston Magazine*, and *Elegant Wedding*, and was voted the Best Facialist in 2004 by the *Improper Bostonian*. She has also been featured as a guest esthetician on *Chronicle*, *A Makeover Story*, *Extreme Makeover*, and *Made* on MTV.

- **Nelson Chan:** superstar hair colorist at the Estetica Salon in Beverly Hills, Chan's work has appeared on the stars of such shows as *Buffy the Vampire Slayer*, *American Dreams*, *The King of Queens*, and *That 70s Show*. He is also the founder of I.S.H., a professional hair-care company that distributes the coveted Ionic Conditioning Treatment to over one thousand salons in the U.S., Puerto Rico, Canada, and Mexico.

- **Jin Soon Choi:** the owner of two Manhattan nail spas which regularly make *New York* magazine's Best of New York list, Choi's regular clients include Julianne Moore and Sarah Jessica Parker. Her work has been heralded on the pages of *Harper's Bazaar*, *InStyle*, *Marie Claire*, *Elle* (she did Beyonce's nails for a cover), and *Allure*.

- **David Cotteblanche:** star stylist and co-owner of New York City's Red Market Salon and Lounge in the trendy Meatpacking District. Cotteblanche worked as a stylist and trainer at Frédéric Fekkai before recently opening his own salon. His work has appeared on many runways, including Christian Dior, Diane Von Furstenberg, Ralph Lauren, Nicole Miller, and Yohji Yamamoto, as well as on the pages of *Elle*, *Town & Country*, *Playboy*, and *Gotham*.

- **Dee DeLuca-Mattos:** vice president of Avancé Skincare, an education-driven company that offers a highly evolved curative spa system that promotes beauty through wellness.

- **Linda Deslauriers:** founder of Hair Garden, a holistic hair company based in Hawaii and Los Angeles, and the author of an upcoming hair-care book.

- **Jeffrey Dover, MD:** top dermatologist, professor, and skin-care entrepreneur. Dr. Dover graduated magna cum laude with an M.D. from the University of Ottawa. He is associate clinical professor of dermatology at Yale University School of Medicine, and adjunct professor of medicine (dermatology) at Dartmouth Medical School. Dr. Dover is a director of SkinCare Physicians in Chestnut Hill, Mass. He is the author of over three hundred published articles and has coauthored/edited seventeen textbooks. He has also recently developed Skin Effects, the first dermatologist-developed anti-aging line for the mass market, for CVS.

- **Manana Dzhanimanova**: senior eyebrow designer at Frédéric Fekkai Salon & Spa in New York City. A native of the Eastern European country of Georgia, Dzhanimanova's career has encompassed stints at top New York salons, including John Barrett at Bergdorf Goodman. Her talent has won her legions of celebrity fans, including Faith Evans, Suzanne Vega, and Lorraine Bracco.

- **Mala Elhassan:** multitasking miracle-worker who triples as a stylist, colorist, and makeup artist at New York City's hip Robert Kree salon.

- **Elisa Ferri:** celebrity manicurist affiliated with Nailene nail-care products. Ferri's work appears regularly in magazines such as *Vogue* and *Allure*, and she is also the coauthor of *Style on Hand: Perfect Nail and Skincare.*

- **Todd Fox:** top colorist at the Frédéric Fekkai Salon & Spa, New York City. Fox received extensive training with L'Oreal, including working under the guidance of Constance Hartnett and a stint on L'Oreal's National Show team. Fox is known for his expertise with corrective color, foil highlights, and his ability to color ethnic hair.

- **Rebecca James Gadberry:** the professional skin-care industry's leading ingredient expert. Gadberry is president and chairman of the board of YG Laboratories, as well as an award-winning journalist, licensed esthetician, and one of the industry's most dynamic educators. Gadberry has been the instructor and sole coordinator for UCLA Extension's highly respected Cosmetic Sciences program since 1986. She has published well over five hundred articles in industry and consumer magazines throughout the world, including *Glamour, Self, Cosmopolitan,* and the *New York Times.* Her insights into cosmetic ingredients have been quoted by such publications as *Shape, Redbook, Essence,* and *Allure.*

- **Diane Gardner:** Hollywood hairstylist, colorist, and makeup artist known as the Makeover Specialist. Drawing on her background working with legendary colorist Louis Licari and makeup artist Trish McEvoy, Gardner offers comprehensive makeovers to entertainment-industry insiders, brides, and everyday men and women from her studio in Los Angeles. She has appeared on *Fashion Emergency* and *Movie and a Makeover*, and her work has appeared on runways and magazine covers.

- **Giella:** professional makeup artist and founder of GIELLA Custom Blend Cosmetics, a custom makeup line sold at Henri Bendel, online, and at salons throughout the East Coast.

- **Fabrice Gili:** hair designer at Frédéric Fekkai Salon & Spa, New York City.

- **Hara Glick:** founder of makeupalley.com, the leading consumer beauty-product review website.

- **Meredith Green:** publicist and lifestyle expert.

- **Dennis Gross, MD:** Manhattan-based dermatologist, creator of MD Skincare, and author of *Your Future Face*. He received his medical degree from New York University Medical Center and began his career as a skin-cancer research scientist. He is currently affiliated with NYU Medical Center.

- **Skyy Hadley:** formerly a top manicurist at posh spots such as the Bliss Spa and the Prive Salon, Hadley is the creator of the As "U" Wish Nail Spa in Hoboken, New Jersey. Her clients include Faith Evans, Uma Thurman, Sean "Diddy" Combs, Liv Tyler, Mariska Hargitay, Alicia Keys, Kelly Rowland, and Chris Webber.

- **Nathaniel Hawkins:** one of New York's premier young hair talents, Hawkins got his start at New York City's Garren Salon in Henri Bendel. Hawkins's celebrity fans include Winona Ryder, Gisele Bündchen, Heidi Klum, Kelly Ripa, Maggie Gyllenhaal, Marcia Cross, Hilary Duff, and Cynthia Nixon. He has worked with the world's top photographers, including Annie Leibovitz, Stephen Meisel, and Patrick Demarchelier, and his work has appeared on the pages of *Vogue*, *W*, *Allure*, *Harper's Bazaar*, and *Elle*. Other clients have included Marc Jacobs, Valentino, Versace, Saks Fifth Avenue, Abercrombie & Fitch, and Lilly Pulitzer. Hawkins is also a spokesperson for TRESemmé Professional European Hair Care.

- **Julie Hewett:** top movie makeup artist for films such as *Pearl Harbor*, *American Beauty*, *Spiderman*, and *Ocean's 11* and *Ocean's 12*, and creator of a bestselling eponymous makeup line.

- **Bettijo B. Hirschi:** creator of Bath By Bettijo, a line of natural, handmade bath and body products that have been featured on the pages of *O*, *Allure*, and *Lucky*.

- **June Jacobs:** skin-care expert, beauty entrepreneur, and founder of June Jacobs Spa Collection.

- **Bobbe Joy:** Lucy Liu, Scarlett Johansson, Naomi Watts, Jennifer Tilly, and Janice Dickinson have put their best face forward with the help of Bobbe Joy, who opened her elegant, private makeup studio in Beverly Hills in 1998. Her signature line of products, Makeup! Bobbe Joy, allows women to create a look which is sophisticated, sensual, and polished.

- **John Ivey, DMD:** celebrity cosmetic dentist practicing in Beverly Hills. Known as the Smile Maker, Ivey's A-list clients include Sharon Stone, Kim Delaney, and Damon Wayans.

- **Peter Lamas:** founder and chairman of Lamas Beauty International, a rapidly growing, well-respected natural beauty–product manufacturer. A beauty industry fixture for more than thirty years, Lamas began his career at Vidal Sassoon and Paul Mitchell. Lamas lectures internationally, and his mastery of hair care, skin care, and makeup has earned him an impressive celebrity following.

- **Jennifer Leung:** owner and founder of the Lavande Nail Spas in San Francisco, Leung's retreats have been voted the best in the city. Leung's goal is to offer the luxury of an exclusive spa at a far more relaxing price.

- **Rachel Lindy:** stylist at Los Angeles's Trim Salon and winner of *Allure*'s coveted Up and Coming Star Stylist award.

- **Fiona Locke:** senior spray technician, California Tan Sunless Spray Tanning System. Fans of California Tan include Britney Spears, Jessica Simpson, Gisele Bündchen, and Hilary Swank.

- **Jerome Lordet:** star stylist at NYC's Pierre Michel Salon. The French native boasts over sixteen years of experience in the beauty industry. His work has graced the heads of celebs like Sandra Bullock and Rebecca Gayheart. Regular clients include Bianca Jagger, Oksana Baiul, and Raquel Welch.

- **Debra B. Luftman, MD:** a Los Angeles–based cosmetic dermatologist. Luftman teaches general dermatology and skin surgery at UCLA and Sepulveda VA hospitals. Dr. Luftman has been featured in many national magazines as well as television programs like *20/20*, *Extra!*, and the Lifetime Television program *New Attitudes*.

- **Mary Lupo, MD:** one of the foremost dermatologists practicing today, Dr. Lupo maintains a successful private practice while also serving as a professor of dermatology at Tulane University Medical School. She has appeared as a skin-care expert on *The View*, E! Entertainment Television, and CNN, and has been featured in every major women's magazine, including *Elle*, *Allure*, *Vogue*, *W*, *Glamour*, and *Self*. Dr. Lupo has also developed a line of eponymous skin-care products.

- **Debra Macki:** a top Boston-based makeup artist, Macki offers classes for professional makeup artists and employs a roster of top makeup artists nationwide. Macki is also the founder of Debra Macki Cosmetics, and her work has been featured in *Vogue, Modern Bride*, *Elegant Wedding*, and *Boston Magazine*.

- **Jan Marini:** skin-care authority, lecturer, product researcher, glycolic acid pioneer, and founder of a highly regarded skin-care line, Jan Marini Skin Research.

- **Damien Miano:** celebrity hairstylist whose work has appeared in countless top magazines, including *Cosmopolitan*, *Glamour*, and *W*. Miano is the co-owner of New York City's hot Miano Viél Salon.

- **Jim Miller:** founder of California North, a West Coast skin-care line.

- **Beth Minardi:** one of America's leading hair color authorities, and co-owner, with husband Carmine, of New York City's Minardi Salon. Dubbed the Highlight Diva by *Glamour* magazine, Minardi has consulted and developed products for the likes of Clairol and Redken. She is responsible for Rene Russo's scene-stealing color in *The Thomas Crowne Affair*, and counts celebrities like Cameron Diaz, Christie Brinkley, Faye Dunaway, Brad Pitt, Matt Dillon, Sarah Jessica Parker, and Mandy Moore among her clients.

- **Angela Nice:** skin-care specialist and creator and cofounder of Los Angeles's M Aesthetics Spa, which is quickly becoming the "body-contouring mecca of L.A." Nice is one of the foremost experts in body sculpting and cellulite reduction (*Allure* dubbed her the Endermologie Guru). She is also a trained electrologist, massage therapist, and esthetician. Her expertise extends to microdermabrasion, acne recovery, cryotherapy, and ultrasound.

- **Rick Noodleman, MD:** cosmetic dermatologist and medical director of Age Defying Dermatology, the largest cosmetic surgery medical center in Silicon Valley. Dr. Noodleman and his wife, Dr. Arlene Noodleman, are the creators of Revercel anti-aging skin-care products.

- **Gabrielle Ophals:** cofounder and co-owner, with Audra Senkus, of Haven Spa, a serene spot in New York City's hip SoHo neighborhood. Haven is regularly featured in *Allure* for its top-notch facials and waxing services.

- **Oribe:** one of the most innovative hairstylists of our time, whose work has dominated the fashion and editorial worlds for sixteen years. Oribe's work has appeared in countless publications, including four hundred covers for magazines such as *Vogue*, *Elle*, and *Harper's Bazaar*. Oribe was the first American hairstylist to do the couture shows in Paris and Milan, and he has worked with countless celebrities, including Jennifer Lopez, Minnie Driver, Andie MacDowell, and Penelope Cruz. Oribe has a signature salon in Miami, and he's the only contemporary stylist to have a permanent exhibit at the Metropolitan Museum of Art.

- **Michelle Ornstein:** owner/founder of Enessa Wellness Spa and its accompanying aromatherapeutic skin-care line. Clients include Jennifer Aniston, Brad Pitt, and Courteney Cox Arquette.

- **Michael O'Rourke:** master hairstylist and founder of Sexy Hair Concepts. O'Rourke is a popular figure on the talk-show circuit, including *Extreme Makeover* and *Soap Talk*. His products are favorites among Hollywood's top stylists, including the experts behind *The O.C.*, *Desperate Housewives*, *Pirates of the Caribbean*, and *Charlie's Angels 2*.

- **Ouidad:** stylist, salon owner, educator, and author who has earned a respected reputation as the Curly Hair Expert. In 1982, Ouidad opened the first salon specializing in curly hair. As a curly-haired woman herself, Ouidad understands the special needs of this often misunderstood and mistreated hair type. This understanding led her to develop an eponymous line of high-quality products designed to specifically address the needs of curly hair.

- **Dee Pearn:** celebrity manicurist with the Artists by Timothy Priano agency. Pearn's work has appeared in countless magazines, including *Vogue*, *Cosmopolitan*, *Elle*, *W*, *Glamour*, *Harper's Bazaar*, *Allure*, *InStyle*, and *Essence*, as well as advertisements for Roca-Wear, Gillette, and H&M. She has also done catalog work for Saks Fifth Avenue, Neiman Marcus, and Victoria's Secret. Her celebrity clients include Mariah Carey, Ashanti, Venus Williams, Catherine Zeta-Jones, Gisele Bündchen, Heidi Klum, Penelope Cruz, Salma Hayek, and Lauryn Hill. Pearn divides her time between Miami, Nantucket, and Europe.

- **Napoleon Perdis:** Australian celebrity makeup artist with an eponymous makeup line. Perdis has worked on famous faces like Alanis Morissette, Cameron Diaz, Drew Barrymore, Gabrielle Union, Janet Jackson, Kylie Minogue, Liv Tyler, Lucy Liu, Naomi Watts, Nicole Kidman, Nicolette Sheridan, Paris Hilton, and Elle MacPherson. His popular makeup line has recently landed stateside at Saks Fifth Avenue.

- **Ric Pipino:** Australian-born stylist with an eponymous hair-care line and salons in New York City, Miami, and Los Angeles. Pipino's work has been featured on the runways of Victoria's Secret, Esteban Cortazar, Ralph Lauren, and Donna Karan and on the pages of *Vogue*, *Elle*, *Glamour*, and *GQ*. Pipino's celebrity clients include Donna Karan, Sarah Wynter, Allison Janney, and Naomi Campbell, and he had a cameo as Ben Stiller's stylist in *Zoolander*.

- **Shauna Raisch:** founder and owner of Twiggs Salonspa of Wayzata, a 3,700-square-foot high-end facility in the Twin Cities. Raisch is a third-generation stylist/salon owner with over nineteen years of experience in the industry. Her skill is in customizing a look for her clients by combining face shape, body shape, color, texture, personal preferences, and maintenance requirements.

- **Diane Ranger:** founder of mineral makeup, and the founder and owner of Colorescience Cosmetics. Ranger founded and developed Bare Escentuals, the first mineral makeup line, twenty-eight years ago, and has since gone on to develop Colorescience, a mineral makeup line that uses only color derived from nature.

- **Barry Reitman:** star hairstylist with over twenty-five years of experience serving an exclusive clientele of celebrities and royalty. His work has been widely featured on television and film, and in magazines such as *Marie Claire* and *L.A. Confidential*.

- **Reynald Ricard:** top colorist whose career began in Paris with the likes of Maniatis, Frank Provot, and Jacques Dessange. His work for Jacques Dessange included assisting with the opening of salons in Casablanca, Paris, and Miami. Ricard's career then took him to New York, where he was a stylist and trainer with Frédéric Fekkai before moving to the prestigious Pierre Michel Salon. He is now the co-owner of the trendy Red Market Salon and Lounge in New York City. He has worked with celebrities like Anne Heche and Sting.

- **Lilly Rivera:** celebrated makeup artist at the prestigious Dominique Salon in the Hotel Pierre, New York City. Rivera has more than twenty years experience in the beauty and bridal industries, and her clients include celebrated beauties such as Lauren Bush, Patricia Duff, Anh Duong, Rachel Hunter, and Amanda Hearst.

- **Anthony Rocanello:** senior colorist at Madison Avenue's Julien Farel Salon in New York City.

- **Peter Thomas Roth:** skin-care entrepreneur and founder of a bestselling eponymous skin-care line.

- **Fabien Roussel:** top New York City stylist with the Julien Farel Salon. Roussel owned a salon in his native France before relocating to the United States. His work has appeared in *Allure*, *Bride's*, *Elle Décor*, *Glamour*, and *Harper's Bazaar*.

- **Anastasia Soare:** dubbed the Eyebrow Queen, Soare's work has graced the world's most famous faces, including those of Madonna, Jennifer Lopez, Renee Zellweger, Debra Messing, Oprah Winfrey, Penelope Cruz, and Reese Witherspoon. Her work has been applauded in such magazines as *Vogue*, *W*, *Town & Country*, *Elle*, *InStyle*, *Allure*, *Entertainment Weekly*, *People*, and *Newsweek*.

- **Kattia Solano:** owner of the hip Butterfly Studio in New York City, which has been featured in Daily Candy (a hip website/email newsletter that has become an authority on trends) and *Allure*. Butterfly Studio is New York City's flagship Kerastase salon, and Solano, formerly of the John Barrett salon, is an expert stylist.

- **Stephen Sollitto:** one of the most sought-after makeup artists in the industry, Sollitto was snatched up by Christina Aguilera as her personal makeup maestro right after her career began. He has also painted the faces of celebs such as Rosario Dawson, Jewel, Erika Christensen, Tara Reid, Shannon Elizabeth, Carmen Electra, and Brooke Burns. His work has been featured in celebrity photo spreads for magazines such as *Vogue*, *Vanity Fair*, *Interview*, *Esquire*, and *InStyle*.

- **Galit Strugano:** makeup artist and creator of Girlactik Beauty, a top-selling makeup line. Strugano's initial concept, to create a glitter makeup that stays put, evolved into an entire line that has become a favorite of celebrities such as Britney

Spears, Carmen Electra, Alicia Keys, Christina Aguilera, Eve, Julia Roberts, and Ali Landry.

- **Vanessa Talabac:** senior esthetician, Le Salon Chinois, New York City, and a skin-care veteran with over fifteen years of experience.

- **Meg Thompson:** Hollywood makeup artist and co-owner and founder, with sister Katherine Thompson and friend Karen Wood, of Madge Cosmetics. The focus of Madge is to inspire and empower women of all ages. Their first line, Elements by Madge, was designed to help teens enhance their natural beauty and to foster self-esteem, character, and charm.

- **Jessica Tingley:** hair designer at Frédéric Fekkai Salon & Spa in Beverly Hills. With fifteen years of experience, Tingley specializes in sexy, long hair. Her work has graced celebrities such as Daisy Fuentes, Maggie Gyllenhaal, Mischa Barton, and Kerry Washington.

- **Jimmy Vanegas:** founder and owner of Beauty Now Management. After graduating from the Fashion Institute of Technology, Vanegas spent years in the salon and spa industries, including the prestigious Frédéric Fekkai Salon. When former Fekkai superstylist Julien Farel left to open his own salon, Vanegas was brought on to manage and market what is now one of the hottest salons in New York City. Vanegas has worked on photo shoots and fashion shows with legendary stylists like Ric Pipino and John Barrett. Beauty Now Management provides public relations and consulting services to a variety of prestigious salon clients.

- **Jessica Vartoughian:** dubbed the First Lady of Nails by the *New York Times*, Vartoughian is Hollywood's leading natural nail–care specialist. In 1969, she opened Jessica Nail Clinic, the first nails-only salon in the country, and soon luminaries like Ronald and Nancy Reagan were paying her regular visits. During the Reagan presidency, she set up a salon in the White House and flew from L.A. to D.C. every other week to attend to the nails of the First Couple. Today, as founder and CEO of Jessica Cosmetics, she has developed an extensive nail-care and color line. Vartoughian is a pioneer who invented the French manicure and was the first to use heated mittens and booties during manicures and pedicures. She is even credited with helping Princess Diana overcome her nail-biting habit. Her current celebrity clients include dozens of Hollywood's top names, including Renee Zellweger, Ashton Kutcher, Jessica Alba, Jessica Simpson, Jodie Foster, Kate Beckinsale, Madonna, Naomi Watts, Reese Witherspoon, Sarah Jessica Parker, and Scarlett Johansson.

- **Louis Viél:** a passionate hair colorist and co-owner of Manhattan's Miano Viél Salon. Viél is a recognized expert in the hair-care industry, having consulted for Helene Curtis and Revlon. His celebrity client list is extensive, and includes Heidi Klum, Melanie Griffith, Melina Kanakaredes, George Stephanopoulos, Tipper Gore, and Karenna Gore Schiff.

- **Charles Worthington:** co-owner and creative director of Charles Worthington salons, with five locations in London and one in New York City, which attract celebrities like Mena Suvari and Jennifer Love Hewitt. Worthington is also the founder of an eponymous hair-care line sold in drugstores worldwide.

- **Hollis Wright:** makeup artist and skin-care expert with over twenty years of experience. Wright's specialty is translating current makeup trends into wearable looks for her varied clientele, who range in age from eleven to eighty-five. Wright's expertise can currently be enlisted at the Sanctuary Salon and Day Spa in Houston. She also serves as a national educator for Colorescience Mineral Makeup.

- **Jessica Wu, MD:** a graduate of Harvard Medical School, dermatologist Dr. Wu is a well-known media personality. She has been featured on *Inside Edition, Extra!*, E! Entertainment Television, FOXNews, and Lifetime. An expert at combining Western science with Chinese medicine, Dr. Wu has appeared on the pages of *Elle*, *InStyle*, *Glamour*, *US Weekly*, and *Cosmopolitan*. In addition to teaching at USC Medical Center and maintaining a private practice, Dr. Wu has also developed her own skin-care line, Dr. Jessica Wu Cosmeceuticals.

- **Wende Zomnir:** creative director of Hard Candy Cosmetics and founder/creative director of Urban Decay Cosmetics.

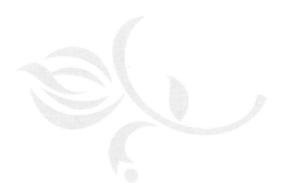

Chapter One

Starworthy Skin Care:
Skin-Saving Strategies Designed to Make Any Woman Spotlight-Ready

"Halle Berry's skin is her best accessory." I read that in a magazine once, and I've never forgotten it. The most beautiful, head-turning, heart-stopping women in the world all have one thing in common: gorgeous, radiant skin. When your skin is healthy and vibrant, it's like a light switch has been turned on inside of you, and the world is drawn to that light. Halle isn't the only celebrity whose glow eclipses her gowns: Jennifer Lopez, Rosario Dawson, Eva Mendes, Scarlett Johansson, and Jennifer Aniston are all known as much for their skin as they are for their style. But you don't need to be a celebrity to make a statement with your skin. Even if you think your complexion is beyond repair, a few of the simple strategies on the following pages can help make it paparazzi-worthy in very little time.

THE *Beauty Bunch* BREAKDOWN

Peter Thomas Roth: skin-care entrepreneur with an eponymous skin-care line.

Jan Marini: skin-care authority and founder of Jan Marini Skin Research.

Jeffrey Dover, MD: top dermatologist, professor, and creator of Skin Effects, the first dermatologist-developed anti-aging line for the mass market.

Giella: professional makeup artist and founder of GIELLA Custom Blend Cosmetics.

Shan Albert: the director of education and product development for Zed Laboratories, the world's leader for revolutionary advances in skin care.

Jessica Wu, MD: Harvard-educated dermatologist and well-known media personality.

Dennis Gross, MD: Manhattan-based dermatologist, creator of MD Skincare, and author of *Your Future Face*.

Danielle Browning: spa director of Boston's famed G Spa.

Mary Lupo, MD: one of the country's foremost dermatologists, Dr. Lupo is also a professor at Tulane University Medical School, a frequent television personality, and a skin-care entrepreneur.

June Jacobs: skin-care expert, beauty entrepreneur, and founder of June Jacobs Spa Collection.

Kathryn Alice: beauty publicist with her own firm, the Alice Company.

Dee DeLuca-Mattos: vice president of Avancé Skincare.

Rebecca James Gadberry: the professional skin-care industry's leading ingredient expert.

REMARKABLE SKIN-CARE REGIMENS

The Buzz from the Beauty Editor

I think it's easy to go to extremes when approaching a skin-care routine, and I'm definitely guilty of this. Either I construct elaborate, impossible daily regimens involving countless products and dozens of steps, or I skip it all entirely and go to sleep with my makeup on. I've found that the answer lies somewhere in the middle. Product overload isn't healthy for your skin, your budget, or your schedule, and neglected skin looks, well, neglected. Find a simple, effective routine that you can stick with, and be consistent. Do it religiously, morning and night, and soon it will become a habit, like brushing your teeth. The following routines will help you get started. Pick one and try it exactly as prescribed, or pick just what works for you and your lifestyle. No matter what you choose, your skin will thank you for it.

Insider Information from the Beauty Bunch

Simple Acne Agenda

"Here's a simple plan for acne: start with a cleanser specially designed for problem skin, like my Beta Hydroxy Acid 2% Acne Wash. Then use a medicated gel with alpha and beta hydroxy acids or ten percent benzoyl peroxide, whichever works better for you (try Peter Thomas Roth AHA-BHA Acne Clearing Gel or BPO Gel 10%). You may need to try both to see what works best. Finish with an anti-shine product to keep oil in check. A good anti-shine product, like Max Anti Shine Mattifying Gel, can go on under or over your makeup, and will leave your skin feeling silky-soft and moisturized. It should absorb oil all day long and sink into your pores to minimize them. It's a must-have." Peter Thomas Roth

Anti-Aging / Anti-Acne Routine

"Start with a cleanser. Work it in first while the skin is still dry, and then use a little water if you want to. Then take a clean washcloth and use it to remove the cleanser and provide mild exfoliation without being abrasive. Splash your face ten to fifteen times with tepid (lukewarm) water. Apply a lipid-soluble vitamin-C serum over your entire face, your neck, and behind your neck and ears. Then use the Jan Marini Skin Research Bioclear Lotion or Cream, Age Intervention Serum or Cream, or Transformation Cream, and Antioxidant Daily Face Protector SPF 30. At night, do the same thing, but replace the sunscreen with benzoyl peroxide. Apply benzoyl peroxide over the other products only to the areas where breakouts tend to occur." Jan Marini

Dry Skin Dos

"You should only wash your face one time per day—before going to bed. Don't wash your face with cleanser in the morning. Just use room temperature tap water and a toner and moisturizer five minutes before applying makeup. The natural secretions from the night before are good for your skin. Think of it as natural moisturizer. Drink lots of water and eat well. Use a night cream. A glycolic-based cream is great for fine lines, wrinkles, and hydration, and so is a vitamin-C serum for rejuvenating cells." Giella

Treating Adult Acne

"There are many topical and systemic treatments for adult acne. The regimen includes cleansing twice daily, use of topical antibiotics, retinoids, and benzoyl peroxide, and if needed, systemic antibiotics may be added. Accutane is extraordinarily helpful for severe acne." Jeffrey Dover, MD

Attack Aging

"For anti-aging, I recommend using a good gentle exfoliating cleanser like my Anti-Aging Cleansing Gel, an eye cream, and a multipurpose anti-aging cream with peptides, like my Mega Rich Intensive Anti-Aging Cellular Repair. A good anti-aging cream or serum, like Unwrinkle, may be expensive, but it's one simple step. Then use a moisturizer with sunscreen during the day. That's a basic routine. On top

of that you can add a toner, a scrub three times a week—Botanical Buffing Beads is a must-have—and a mask once a week. I usually recommend two eye creams, like Peter Thomas Roth Mega Rich Intensive Anti-Aging Cellular Eye Creme twice a day and Peter Thomas Roth Power K Eye Rescue underneath at night. Add a lightener, like my Potent Skin Lightening Gel Complex, if you need it, to fade spots, and always follow with sunscreen during the day. Don't forget to put sunscreen on your décolleté area and on your hands. Many people can actually do their entire skin-care routine on those areas, but be careful: the skin on the neck and décolleté area is thinner and can be more sensitive, so patch test it first." Peter Thomas Roth

KINDER, GENTLER SKIN CARE

The Buzz from the Beauty Editor

I have been blessed with resilient skin. Nothing irritates it. I remember sitting in the office of a prominent Miami dermatologist and witnessing his amazement as a 70 percent glycolic-acid peel failed to make my skin flush. He left it on far longer than the typically allotted time, and yet my skin showed no signs of distress. I used to think that the absence of sensitive signs, such as redness, dryness, and irritation, meant that my skin could take anything, and that's simply not true. It's not just the sensitive types that need to proceed with caution. We all have sensitive skin, to varying degrees, and if the damage doesn't show up as redness now, it can show up as premature aging later. Skin-care abuse and product overuse shows up on everyone eventually. Your skin is fragile and vulnerable. Treat it that way.

Insider Information from the Beauty Bunch

Take It Easy on Your Skin

"It is important to remember that you need to be kind to the skin and avoid irritating it or causing inflammation. Do not vigorously rub or massage active ingredients into the skin—even natural botanicals or essential oils. Scrubs, if used at all, should be used with a gentle hand. Also, the public is so used to products that do nothing that they think nothing of misusing or overusing a product. If a product contains high enough percentages of active ingredients to be truly effective, then it is possible to have an adverse reaction if the product is misused or overused." Shan Albert

Pare Down the Products

"Being too aggressive and putting too many products on your skin are the most common mistakes. People will use vitamin C followed by an AHA in the morning, and then a scrub followed by Retin-A in the evening, and then they wake up all irritated and red and wonder what's wrong with their skin." Jessica Wu, MD

Multitasking Products

"I believe it is in the consumer's best interests to use one product for multiple purposes. I like to consolidate, not proliferate. If you look at the ingredient list of any skin-care product, the last four to six ingredients are there for shelf life: preservatives, emulsifiers, and chemicals that are necessary, but their use should be minimized if possible. If you use a product that has three [key ingredients] in one, you've cut down on the chemicals. It gives you better skin over time." Dennis Gross, MD

Reducing Redness

"Redness can be caused by a few things—dryness, irritation, or a skin disorder. If you are not using a moisturizer or if your moisturizer is too light, your skin might be 'thirsty.' Also, take notice of any new products that you are using on your face, a new detergent, or any hormonal changes. If you have not tried anything new and are not going through any hormonal changes, then you can check with a dermatologist. There are topical lotions/creams that will help calm the skin and treat such skin conditions. Using a concealer under foundation can hide redness." Giella

Acne and Aggression

"All too often, products made to clear acne contain ingredients to dry up the oil and aggressively exfoliate. I believe in treating an acneic skin gently—not being too aggressive. Why? Because a too-aggressive approach can aggravate the problem. Think about this: the body produces oil on the skin for protection. If the skin becomes irritated or too dry, the skin will send messages to the oil-producing glands to send up more oil. Also, irritation and inflammation can cause premature aging. I would avoid products containing acetone (commonly used as nail-polish remover). This is placed in products to dry up the oil." Shan Albert

USING YOUR PRODUCTS

The Buzz from the Beauty Editor
Choosing the right products is only the first step. Learning how to use them is equally important. From the order of application to specific application techniques, the tips that follow will help you make the most of the time and money that you spend on your skin-care routine.

Insider Information from the Beauty Bunch

Application Order
When applying multiple skin-care products, use the "product with the fastest penetration first, usually the lightest one. So start with liquids, then gels, then lotions, then creams, then ointments. Otherwise, the heavier ones can prevent the penetration of the lighter ones. Sunscreen can be applied at any step in your skin-care routine, according to how heavy or light it is." Dennis Gross, MD

Retinoic Relief
"The best way to use retinoic acid is to apply it in a pea-sized drop divided by four and applied to the dry face every second or third night, and eventually increase to every night or every second night. Retinol does not work nearly as well as tretinoin, which is the other name for retinoic acid. Retinoic acid is available by prescription only and retinol is available over-the-counter, and it is important not to confuse the two and not to assume that retinol will give the results of retinoic acid." Jeffrey Dover, MD

Toner Tips
"If you rinse very well, you do not necessarily need a toner. However, I usually recommend one. It takes off extra traces of cleanser and disinfects the skin from tap water. It also gives you extra benefits from the ingredients, such as aloe, chamomile, and vitamins. It 'prepares' the skin for a moisturizer, and last but not least, it feels good." Giella

Night and Day
"Most people do not realize that you should never use a facial moisturizer with an SPF on your skin at night. Moisturizers with an SPF work differently than moisturizers without sunblock. They are designed to sit on the surface of your skin and prevent your own natural moisture from escaping. A moisturizer without SPF can actually penetrate the surface layers of the skin and affect changes in hydration levels, plump fine lines, et cetera. So both are actually crucial to well-balanced skin." Danielle Browning

MINIMUM PRODUCTS, MAXIMUM BENEFITS

The Buzz from the Beauty Editor
Some mornings, let's face it: it's all we can do to splash water on our faces and stumble out the door. On days like this, I am thankful for the new multi-ingredient skin-care treatment creams. After cleansing my face, I smooth on my anti-aging treatment under my sunscreen, and I'm done. This way, even on the laziest days my skin is always protected and never naked.

Insider Information from the Beauty Bunch

The Three Products Every Woman Needs

"A sunscreen, a retinoid, and an antioxidant are the three skin-care products that every woman needs. Take your pick of antioxidants. Prevage, vitamin C, and flavonoids like grapeseed extract are my favorites." Mary Lupo, MD

Skin Care for Beginners

"Your skin-care routine should depend on what you are trying to achieve with your skin. All women can learn to become their own skin-care expert and consistency is the way you see results. For a basic skin-care routine, start with a cleanser, followed by a treatment, and then a moisturizer applied morning and night. In the morning, make sure your moisturizer has an SPF of at least fifteen, preferably thirty. Treatment products can include serums with high concentrations of antioxidants that promote cell turnover and help prevent wrinkles and fine lines from forming. There are treatment products that help rosacea, adult or teenage acne, hyperpigmentation, and wrinkles. These three steps are all you need to be on your way to having beautiful skin. I don't think you need to overload yourself with tons of products to get results. People get discouraged if you throw too much at them; I remember how I was when I was first exposed to skin care." June Jacobs

Sleepy Solution

"Too tired or lazy to take your makeup off at night? Keep disposable makeup-remover towels, the kind that looks like baby wipes, next to your bed for a quick and easy face wash." Kathryn Alice

THE SKIN/DIET CONNECTION

The Buzz from the Beauty Editor

There is no established link between diet and skin, but that doesn't mean that what you eat doesn't play a part in how you look. It simply means that it's a very individual thing. There is no single food, for example, that will trigger acne in everyone. My skin seems to glow when I eat a lot of fruit, and look lackluster after a fast-food binge. Whether you've noticed similar reactions or not, one thing is certain: diet is critical to your overall health, and skin is an outward reflection of that inward health and vitality. Feed it well.

Insider Information from the Beauty Bunch

Food for Thought

"Diet is important [to skin], but within reason. Eating blueberries will not get rid of wrinkles, but a diet high in such antioxidants is part of a comprehensive, healthy lifestyle that reduces cancer and heart disease and slows aging." Mary Lupo, MD

The Supplement Myth

"There is no evidence that dietary supplementation helps to prevent aging, but this has not stopped a burgeoning multimillion-dollar industry from developing. Eating a balanced diet rich in vegetables, fruits, and essential oils is critical to good skin. Also, exercising regularly and sleeping sufficiently is essential for good skin." Jeffrey Dover, MD

Acne and Diet

"There is definitely a lot more adult acne these days, but no one knows the reason for it. Asians living in Asia have less acne, for some reason. Even though there's no definite proof of a diet link, a lot of my patients see a connection to diet. So I tell them, if you think there's a certain food that makes you break out, by all means, stop eating it." Jessica Wu, MD

TREATING YOUR NECK, CHEST, AND HANDS

The Buzz from the Beauty Editor

I've always continued my skin-care routine down to my neck. It just seemed to make sense. Recently, I discovered that this is an effective strategy for warding off a crepey neck. I've also learned that it's important to continue my routine down to my décolleté, as well as the backs of my hands. This way, I'll be able to avoid turning into one of those women we've all seen, with fresh, youthful faces sitting on sagging necks and wrinkled décolleté.

Insider Information from the Beauty Bunch

Not Just for Your Face Anymore

"We recommend anti-aging products applied to the face, neck, and chest as well as to the backs of the hands in the appropriate candidate." Jeffrey Dover, MD

Comprehensive Anti-Aging

"Use the same anti-aging products on your neck, chest, and hands that you do on your face, but if you have brown spots on your chest and hands, they may not respond as quickly because they don't turn over as quickly. You might have to use stronger products. I think the chest can sometimes be a little more sensitive, so sometimes I'll have patients use products more sparingly or just a few times a week on the neck and chest. I don't think that there are products that will firm the skin on the neck better than the face. The only time I think you need to use something different is if one part is more sensitive than the other." Jessica Wu, MD

Neck Care

"Like the face, the neck and chest get a lot of sun exposure and are subject to the same ravages of sun damage. That is why the same products and routine you use on your face are appropriate for your neck and chest. A gentle cleanser, a sunscreen with avobenzone, titanium dioxide or zinc oxide, Retin-A or Renova, a well-formulated AHA product, and a lightweight moisturizer are the best options possible. You do not need any special product that does not help with sun protection." Giella

IS "NATURAL" BETTER?

The Buzz from the Beauty Editor

"Natural" products are a major skin-care trend, and the big cosmetic manufacturers are responding with an influx of products touted as being "natural." The problem is many of these products contain natural ingredients in very small doses, with synthetic bases and preservatives, making any natural value dubious at best. If natural is important to you, look for products from a skin-care company with a commitment to natural ingredients, because these are the companies that know how to process those ingredients to ensure that they retain their potency. Also, look for natural ingredients at the top of an ingredient list. Farther down, and you may not be getting what you're paying for.

Insider Information from the Beauty Bunch

Plant Problems

"Plant extracts should be chemically standardized, but most companies don't preserve the activity in the product. Let's say I was using a chamomile extract. There are several key chemicals in chamomile, depending on whether it's German chamomile or Roman chamomile. In German chamomile, there's a key chemical, bisabolol, which is an antioxidant and a primary calmative agent. If I harvest it but don't protect the activity of the chemical, then in a week or two the ingredient won't be in there. I can put it on the label, but you won't know if it's active or not because you won't know how I handled it. There is no definite expiration date in the U.S., and even if there is, what is the expiration for? Is it for the effectiveness of the ingredients, or for when they start to separate?" Rebecca James Gadberry

Natural Knowledge

"If a company tells you that their products are all plant-based and don't contain any chemicals, that's a pretty good tip-off that they don't know what they are talking about. A product cannot be chemical-free; if it were, it would be a vacuum. The only things that are not chemicals are light and electricity. How do they know to standardize and protect chemicals when they are not even aware that the chemicals are in there? The people who develop products are called cosmetic chemists because they work with chemicals. For example, the most common solvent for plant extracts is propylene glycol, and propylene comes from petroleum. I would doubt very strongly a product that claims to be all-natural. All-natural products need to be kept in the refrigerator and have a short life." Rebecca James Gadberry

Natural or Synthetic

"A chemical is a chemical. Your skin can't tell which chemical is natural and which is synthetic. As we say in chemistry, a molecule is a molecule; it really doesn't matter where it comes from. It may make a difference to the consumer, but not to the skin." Rebecca James Gadberry

DEFEATING DARK CIRCLES

The Buzz from the Beauty Editor

I've always battled dark under-eye circles, and as I get older and lose some of the fullness in my face, they become even more apparent. Unfortunately, dark circles are one of the trickier issues to treat, and even the experts disagree as to the causes and the best courses of treatment. Try some of the solutions explained here to see which works best for you.

Insider Information from the Beauty Bunch

Eye Shadows

"Dark circles are more complicated than they appear. Not all dark circles are created equal. They can be caused by a number of factors, including pigmentation, the sun, genetics, and/or birth control. One of the ways to get dark circles is if the capillaries in the skin become leaky. Blood can be spilled into the skin, and there is iron in the hemoglobin. When iron is leaked to the skin, it imparts a rusty color. Behind the skin, there are fat pads and blood vessels, and as we age and skin becomes thinner and more transparent, you can see through it to the blood vessels, and this makes it look dark. If you have allergies, you need to stay on an antihistamine; you should take it regularly, not only as needed. Excessive alcohol and smoking are also not good. You can combat these problems. My eye products contain vitamin C and genestein to thicken skin, and cucumber extract, caffeine, and vitamin K to help stabilize the blood vessels. Kojic acid also helps, as a lightener. That's the mix of ingredients that can help tackle dark circles." Dennis Gross, MD

Banishing Shadows

"If you have chronic darkness under your eyes, it could mean sinus problems. Get a neti pot and bathe your sinuses once a day in salt water like the Chinese do. This clears up most sinus problems and results in a shadow-free area under your eyes." Kathryn Alice

Causes and Treatments

"Dark under-eye circles are caused by a combination of hyperpigmentation, blue vessels, and redundant skin. These vessels can be treated with long-pulsed Nd:YAG lasers, but only in expert hands. The pigmentation can be treated with Q-switched lasers, again in expert hands. Lightening agents for the most part are not as effective." Jeffrey Dover, MD

DEPUFFING YOUR EYES

The Buzz from the Beauty Editor

Puffiness can be caused by many factors, from age to diet to heredity. Fortunately, there are some temporary solutions. Pick an eye gel instead of a cream, since creams tend to plump skin up, and, since cold constricts, try a cool compress. Read on for more solutions.

Insider Information from the Beauty Bunch

The Causes of Puffiness

"How you treat puffiness depends on the cause. If it's temporary puffiness caused by a night out, put your eye cream in the fridge, and sometimes the coolness can help shrink the tissues. Chilled cucumber slices or tea bags can also help shrink tissue. Sometimes it's fat and it's hereditary, and the only treatment is surgical. The skin in the eye area is so thin, and any fluid trapped in the face will go to the eyes. Avoid salty foods at night and sleep with your head elevated to help fluid drain away from the eyes. And Preparation H really works. Models and actresses use it. One of my nurses went out and purchased a tube and wrote down the ingredients and there is an ingredient in it that reduces inflammation." Jessica Wu, MD

Problems with Puffiness

"The best treatment for lower-lid and upper-lid puffiness which is caused by fat is blepharoplasty [eyelid surgery]. Eyelid puffiness from fluid retention is best treated with diuretics, if necessary, keeping the head elevated while sleeping, and avoiding salt-laden foods." Jeffrey Dover, MD

Puffy Peepers

"Address puffy eyes with cucumber extract and caffeine, which causes constriction of blood vessels. Alcohol doesn't help, and neither does high sodium, particularly during menstruation. Salt and alcohol together in your diet will cause more puffiness, so avoid that." Dennis Gross, MD

GOING FOR THE GLOW

The Buzz from the Beauty Editor

A gorgeous glow is one of the most elusive outward signs of great skin, and it can't be achieved with products alone. The most elaborate skin-care routine won't compensate for poor diet, insufficient sleep, chain-smoking, and other lifestyle factors. A healthy lifestyle is essential to any lasting skin-care benefits. Fortunately, you don't need a flawless lifestyle to improve your outlook. Regular facials, gentle but thorough exfoliation, and a balanced, comprehensive skin-care routine can greatly enhance your glow, whether you're health-conscious or hedonistic.

Insider Information from the Beauty Bunch

Exfoliation Education

"Exfoliation of the skin is most effective when you combine both chemical exfoliants—beta- and alpha hydroxy acids—and physical exfoliants—scrubs—into your weekly routine. Physical exfoliants remove surface dead skin cells, and chemical exfoliants loosen the bond that holds dead skin cells together so that they shed more effectively. Most estheticians combine different types of exfoliants in their facials, and that is what gives your skin that gorgeous 'just had a facial' glow." Danielle Browning

Frequent Facials

"Skin care is about finding out what works for you, in the right combination, and not being afraid to try something new. I recommend getting monthly facials. Problem skin can go more regularly, maybe twice a month. You see results and it's a way of caring for yourself. Beautiful skin reflects a healthy lifestyle. I make it a point to go as frequently as possible." June Jacobs

Washcloth Wonder

"Always cleanse skin with a cotton washcloth. This acts as a natural exfoliator every time you cleanse." Dee DeLuca-Mattos

THE PRODUCT FILES

Cleansers

The Buzz from the Beauty Editor

I look for a water-soluble cleanser that is gentle yet thorough. It gets extra points if it doubles as a makeup remover, since this saves a step and prevents wear and tear on the skin. If I'm wearing a face full of makeup, I smooth my cleanser over my entire face and then let it sit while I do something else, like brush my teeth. This gives the cleanser a chance to do its thing, and the makeup rinses away with minimal effort. Two of my favorite cleansers are Cetaphil Daily Facial Cleanser Normal/Oily Skin, $7, and Yon-Ka Gel Nettoyant, $35.

What the Pros Choose

Choices range from the herbal, like Enessa Lavender Cleanser (Michelle Ornstein) and Bior Sage Milk (Julie Hewett), to the clinical, like DDF (Galit Strugano), Peter Thomas Roth Anti-Aging Cleansing Gel and Peter Thomas Roth Chamomile Cleansing Lotion (Peter Thomas Roth), and Peter Thomas Roth Sensitive Skin Cleansing Gel (Danielle Browning). Others go for spa favorites, like Eve Lom (Mala Elhassan), Haven Daily Cleansing Milk (Gabrielle Ophals), Catherine Atzen AM-PM Cleansing Gel (Vanessa Talabac), June Jacobs Pore Purifying Cleanser (June Jacobs), and Avancé Foaming Cleansing Gel (Dee DeLuca-Mattos). Two pros pick Pevonia: Meg Thompson (Pevonia Phyto-Gel Cleanser) and Shauna Raisch (Pevonia RS2 Rosacea Gentle Cleanser). Budget picks include Cetaphil (Hara Glick) and L'Oreal Pure Zone Gel (Wende Zomnir). The creative-name awards go to Linda Deslauriers's The Vital Image Grime Fighter and Shan Albert's Sircuit Cosmeceuticals X-Trap Daily Gentle Face Wash, which she claims makes a fan of everyone who tries it.

Toners

The Buzz from the Beauty Editor

I know that toners are not considered an essential step, but for me, they're indispensable. No matter how thoroughly I wash my face, I still feel the need to use a toner. I love how fresh and smooth they leave my skin. It's a myth that you should rub a toner-soaked cotton pad over your skin until it comes up clean. After a couple of swipes, the "dirt" on the cotton pad is not dirt at all; it is dead skin cells that are being exfoliated. One quick swipe with toner is enough; too many may leave skin raw and overexfoliated. My favorites are Yon-Ka Lotion PG Toner, $26, Neutrogena Alcohol-Free Toner, $7, and Fresh Bergamot Anise Tonic Water, $28.

What the Pros Choose

The choices range from floral fixes like Amanda Lacey Persian Rosewater (Julie Hewett) and Enessa Neroli Hydrosol (Michelle Ornstein) to old standbys like Sea Breeze (Kathryn Alice) and L'Oreal Pure Zone (Wende Zomnir, who recommends it for oily, acne-prone skin only). Peter Thomas Roth chooses his toners, as does Danielle Browning (who specifies Peter Thomas Roth Oxygen Mist for its ability to kill surface bacteria), and June Jacobs selects her Pore Purifying Toner. Other picks include Dr. Hauschka

Clarifying Toner (Meg Thompson), Aveda Botanical Kinetics Skin Firming/Toning Agent (Shauna Raisch), Catherine Atzen Tonic Lotion (Vanessa Talabac), and Cosmedix Benefit Balance (Shan Albert). Albert has much to say about Cosmedix Benefit Balance: "It's an antioxidant toner with very high percentages of active ingredients such as cassia betaglycan (a plant collagen that calms the skin), shea butter, L-lactic acid (for softening and gentle exfoliation), heavy water (D2O, which is ten percent heavier than regular water, so it doesn't evaporate as quickly, making it a true hydration agent), and vitamin C. Most traditional toners function as a pH restorer or for removing the last traces of debris from the skin. Benefit Balance does quite a bit more."

Scrubs

The Buzz from the Beauty Editor

Scrubs are one of the most misunderstood aspects of skin care. There are two types of exfoliators: chemical (AHAs, for example) and physical (washcloths, skin brushes, or granulated scrubs). Both can be beneficial, but only in moderation. Too much exfoliation leaves skin raw and vulnerable. I choose exfoliants that are effective yet easy on the skin. Grainy scrubs should be handled with care; you don't want to cause microscopic tears in your skin. That's why I use mine near the end of my shower, when skin is moistened. It makes the scrub much gentler and more effective. Also, limit use to three times a week. My favorites are Dermalogica Daily Microfoliant, $41.50, and Skin Effects Purifying Effects Deep-Cleaning Enzyme Scrub, $7.

What the Pros Choose

Top exfoliators range from kitchen staples like baking soda (Hara Glick) and sugar (when combined with The Vital Image Face and Body Wash, it's Linda Deslauriers's pick) to those that simply sound like they were whipped up in the kitchen, like June Jacobs Mandarin Polishing Beads (June Jacobs) and Skingenious Pumpkin-A-Peel (Shan Albert). Other naturally derived products include Aveda Botanical Kinetics Exfoliant (Shauna Raisch), Enessa Bio-Exfoliant (Michelle Ornstein), Boscia Facial Smoothing Polish (Meredith Green), and Peter Thomas Roth Botanical Buffing Beads (Peter Thomas Roth). The remaining picks include Sonya Dakar Triple Action Organic Scrub (the choice of Gabrielle Ophals and Danielle Browning, who loves it because "it's a physical and chemical exfoliant in one!"), Dr. Brandt Microdermabrasion in a Jar (Wende Zomnir), Janet Sartin Papaya Enzyme Scrub (Julie Hewett), and Dermalogica Daily Microfoliant (Vanessa Talabac).

Moisturizers

The Buzz from the Beauty Editor

I am not one of those people who believes that everyone, regardless of skin type, needs a moisturizer. Moisturizers are for dry skin, period. Oily types don't need them. However, now that I'm in my mid-thirties, my formerly greasy complexion has dried out quite a bit, and my skin type has become more combination than oily. I use a moisturizer only as necessary on dry patches, or all over if my skin feels taut. If I want a more natural, daytime look, I apply my foundation immediately after my moisturizer, or cut it with a little moisturizer before applying it. It has almost the same effect as a tinted moisturizer, but with slightly more coverage. For full coverage, I wait a few minutes for the moisturizer to sink in. My favorites are Peter Thomas Roth Oil Free Moisturizer, $40, Awake Hydro-Force Oil Free Treatment, $45, Dermalogica Barrier Repair Cream, $37, and Aveeno Positively Radiant Daily Moisturizer with SPF15, $14.

What the Pros Choose

Our pros pick products on both ends of the price spectrum, from Olay (Kathryn Alice and Hara Glick) to Crème de la Mer (Wende Zomnir). Other favorites include Murad Perfecting Day Serum (Meredith Green), Enessa Seaweed Nourishing Gel (Michelle Ornstein), Prada Beauty Reviving Face Bio-Firm SPF 15 (Meg Thompson), Bior Crème de Beaute (Julie Hewett), June Jacobs Skin Amour Day Cream (June Jacobs), Avancé Potion (Dee DeLuca-Mattos), Catherine Atzen Advanced Bio-Active Complex (Vanessa Talabac), Aveda Tourmaline Charged Hydrating Creme (Shauna Raisch), Sircuit Molecular Mist Hydrating Moisture Care (Shan Albert), and Peter Thomas Roth (Peter Thomas Roth). Gabrielle Ophals has two top picks, Haven Liquid Drench and Yon-Ka Crème 15: "The Crème 15 uses the properties of various essential oils to naturally disinfect. We like to use it post-extraction, and we also recommend it as a moisturizer for people suffering from problem skin." Linda Deslauriers also had more than one favorite: The Vital Image Phytohydrator, The Vital Image Skin Renewal Complex, and Martina Gebhardt Kosmetik Rose Facial Lotion.

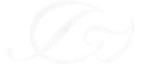

Eye Creams

The Buzz from the Beauty Editor

I've been using eye cream since I was in junior high, and my obsession with my under-eye area has only grown with age. Heredity has blessed me with dark circles, and the constant onslaught of birthdays threatens to produce fine lines. I look for an eye cream that is hydrating yet soothing, absorbs easily, and won't irritate my sensitive eyes. I apply eye cream with my ring finger, and I dab it on—no rubbing. It's the easiest way to ensure that you don't tug at or otherwise injure this delicate area. My favorites are Neutrogena Visibly Firm Eye Cream, $18.50, and Clarins Skin Smoothing Eye Mask, $41.50 (which doubles as a cream).

What the Pros Choose

The pros go for luxury in this category, with choices ranging from La Mer Eye Balm (Julie Hewett) to Cle de Peau Eye Contour Balm (Meg Thompson) to IS Clinical Eye Complex (Vanessa Talabac). Thompson also has a second, more moderately priced pick: Dr. Hauschka Eye Contour Day Balm. June Jacobs chooses her own Firming Eye Cream; Wende Zomnir picks Franché Eye Treat; Meredith Green reaches for Murad Moisture Silk Eye Gel; Hara Glick picks Shiseido Benefiance Eye Cream; Shauna Raisch likes Aveda Tourmaline Charged Eye Crème; Michelle Ornstein sticks with Enessa Rose Oil; Gabrielle Ophals loves Sjal Orbe; Danielle Browning chooses Nature by Valmont Taking Care of Lips and Eyes; Peter Thomas Roth chooses his own Power K Eye Rescue; and Linda Deslauriers goes for The Vital Image Eye Area Builder. Dee DeLuca-Mattos keeps her choice a mystery—she's currently testing a secret eye cream that's become her fave. Shan Albert can't say enough about her pick, Sircuit Cosmeceuticals White Out, which she claims "lightens, brightens, eliminates dark circles, and moisturizes the eye area as it gently exfoliates to reduce the signs of aging around the eye."

Eye Makeup Removers

The Buzz from the Beauty Editor

I don't wear waterproof eye makeup, so my requirements in a makeup remover are that it's gentle enough for my sensitive eyes and that it easily eliminates makeup without rubbing or scrubbing. I prefer to use eye-makeup remover after cleansing, to remove any residue left behind by my face wash. This also prevents excessive rubbing and tugging. My favorites are Lancôme Effacil, $21, and Swabplus Mascara Remover Swabs, $4.

What the Pros Choose

Choices range from Enessa (Michelle Ornstein) to Clinique (Hara Glick), and from Clarins (Julie Hewett) to Peter Thomas Roth Gentle Eye & Face Makeup Remover (Peter Thomas Roth) and June Jacobs Gentle Creamy Eye Makeup Remover (June Jacobs). Other picks include Almay Non-Oily Eye Makeup Remover Pads (Meg Thompson), Sephora Soothing Eye Makeup Remover (Galit Strugano), Avancé Eye Makeup Remover (Dee DeLuca-Mattos), Pevonia Eye Makeup Remover Lotion (Shauna Raisch), and Dermalogica Soothing Eye Makeup Remover (Vanessa Talabac).

Chapter Two

Skin-Care Specifics:
Treating and Beating Your Most Troublesome Skin-Care Issues

We've all seen worst-dressed lists, where style pundits rip the sketchy style of certain celebs to shreds, but I recently came across a worst-skin list. Shockingly, this list included some of the world's most famously gorgeous faces, including Jessica Simpson, Brad Pitt, and, at number one, Cameron Diaz. Now it may be small consolation to know that even the world's most beautiful people suffer from the indignities of acne, but it does show that nobody is above the occasional skin problem. For those of us not blessed with twenty-four-hour makeup crews (and distractions like Cameron's legs or Jessica's curves), problem skin is a threat to our well-being and self-esteem. Fortunately, whether you suffer from blemishes or brown spots, wrinkles or rosacea, the pros on these pages will show you the simplest solutions and the most surefire strategies.

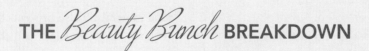

THE *Beauty Bunch* BREAKDOWN

Peter Thomas Roth: skin-care entrepreneur with an eponymous skin-care line.

Jan Marini: skin-care authority and founder of Jan Marini Skin Research.

Jeffrey Dover, MD: top dermatologist, professor, and creator of Skin Effects, the first dermatologist-developed anti-aging line for the mass market.

Giella: professional makeup artist and founder of GIELLA Custom Blend Cosmetics.

Shan Albert: the director of education and product development for Zed Laboratories, the world's leader for revolutionary advances in skin care.

Jessica Wu, MD: Harvard-educated dermatologist and well-known media personality.

Dennis Gross, MD: Manhattan-based dermatologist, creator of MD Skincare, and author of *Your Future Face*.

Mary Lupo, MD: one of the country's foremost dermatologists, Dr. Lupo is also a professor at Tulane University Medical School, a frequent television personality, and a skin-care entrepreneur.

Wende Zomnir: creative director of Hard Candy Cosmetics and founder/creative director of Urban Decay Cosmetics.

Rebecca James Gadberry: the professional skin-care industry's leading ingredient expert.

Gabrielle Ophals: cofounder and co-owner of Haven Spa, a serene spot in New York City's hip SoHo neighborhood.

Jim Miller: founder of California North, a West Coast skin-care line.

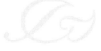

BATTLING BLEMISHES

The Buzz from the Beauty Editor

I was fifteen when my dermatologist told me that my skin would probably clear up by twenty. By then, I thought, I'll be dead. Or too old to care. Looking back, I wish he was right. Acne reared its ugly head for a second time in adulthood, and this time, it was even more complicated. My skin could no longer handle the harsh products and persistent picking I'd subjected it to as a teenager. I still needed to treat acne; I just needed to do it more gently. Fortunately, there are plenty of products and procedures designed to do just that.

Insider Information from the Beauty Bunch

Causes of Acne

"The main causes [of acne] are overproduction of oil, heredity, and hormones. There are other special types of acne, like acne cosmetica, which is caused by the use of cosmetics. In terms of treatment, I can't say that one treatment is best because it depends on the cause. That's why a product like Proactiv, which works for many people, doesn't work for everyone. Monthly breakouts are more than likely hormonal, so a hormonal treatment like the Pill works best. Pustules on the face throughout the month might be bacteria, so antibiotics in the tetracycline family might work." Jessica Wu, MD

The Pimple Pill

"The prescription diuretic spironolactone is a generic medication that's been around for over thirty years and can virtually eliminate adult acne in many cases. It's potassium-sparing, and does not deplete you of good minerals. It also prevents bloating, and decreases cravings for salt, sugar, and chocolate. You can take twenty-five to one hundred and fifty milligrams a day, and it's fairly inexpensive. Some doctors don't know about this, but for women with resistant recalcitrant breakouts, it works so well. It even normalizes the oil in the T zone." Jan Marini

Pore Problems

"Retinoids and Intense Pulsed Light are the best treatments [for problem pores]." Mary Lupo, MD

Smart Squeezing

"Everybody squeezes. No one wants to have blackheads or blemishes on their face. I believe in squeezing gently but doing it the right way. The best way is to cleanse in the shower to soften your skin and open your pores, dry off, gently squeeze, put some of my Sulfur Cooling Mask on after a few minutes to tighten the pores and prevent breakouts, and then use Cucumber Gel Masque afterwards for five to ten minutes to calm the skin. After that, use your acne treatment product. Everything will be open and vulnerable, so you want the medicine to go right in, in case you just triggered some acne." Peter Thomas Roth

Scrub Setback

"I do not believe that scrubs are a good choice as an exfoliant for skin prone to blemishes. Scrubbing an already irritated and inflamed skin is, to my mind, a terrible idea, and it could open the blemishes and spread infection. I much prefer using L-lactic acid or salicylic acid for exfoliation." Shan Albert

Adult-Acne Epidemic

"Adult acne is an epidemic. There's a controversial theory that it may be triggered or exacerbated by a lifetime of consuming refined carbohydrates. A lot of doctors believe it is a contributing factor and there have been some studies pointing to it. One published medical study examined different cultures all over the world, in order to do comparisons between cultures that experience acne and those that don't. The glaring difference was the consumption of refined carbohydrates. The study found that we are consuming higher levels of refined carbohydrates over a lifetime: cereal, pasta, bread, and sweets, et cetera. This, in turn, generates higher insulin levels. Generally, most people deal with it well, but some people become insulin-resistant and it contributes to higher levels of obesity. In a lot of individuals, high inconsistent glucose levels can trigger a mild endocrine imbalance that may contribute to more androgens, such as testosterone. Unfortunately, you can't just stop eating refined carbs and have it go away. It's like thinking that if you stop smoking your cancer will go away." Jan Marini

Smart Buy

"Buy an extractor. It can do search and destroy on surface blemishes and unclog pores that are about to go south. But don't use it on deep pimples." Wende Zomnir [Note: using an extractor on deep pimples can lead to scarring.]

Peels, Explained

"Salicylic-acid peels are the most effective [treatment for acne]. Most of my patients receive a Jessner peel. It's a combination of salicylic acid, which gets into the oil glands and breaks up the clogging, and lactic acid, to help exfoliate. Salicylic acid is also an anti-inflammatory. You can also do a salicylic-acid peel on the chest and back. For aging, the best thing is a TCA peel. It's got about a week of recovery time, but it really helps to relieve fine lines and take off hyperpigmentation. It just looks like you have a sunburn for a week." Jessica Wu, MD

Microdermabrasion for Acne

"Microdermabrasion and gentle glycolic peels help to polish the skin and make it generally look better. They do help some causes of hyperpigmentation, and very mild acne, especially where comedones are frequent." Jeffrey Dover, MD

BEATING BLACKHEADS

The Buzz from the Beauty Editor

A close friend of mine with gorgeous, even-toned skin has a tendency to get blackheads around her nose. Her skin is otherwise flawless, but those stubborn blackheads keep cropping up. The tendency to get blackheads is hereditary, so unfortunately, though a good skin-care routine can minimize them, it probably won't prevent them altogether. The best way to keep them in check is with regular facials, because the only way to remove a blackhead is to extract it, and this is best left to a professional.

Insider Information from the Beauty Bunch

Fight Back with Facials

"Facials are very important for thorough extractions and a deep cleaning to help get rid of blackheads and blemishes in hard-to-reach areas. You can only get to certain areas yourself, so basically at-home squeezing is a temporary fix in between facials. An esthetician can also remove some large blemishes that you would not be able to do yourself. Whenever I get a facial, I always ask the esthetician to concentrate on extractions, extractions, extractions. I love the pampering of a facial, but for me I want everything out in my hour.

"Anti-aging facials are important as well, since the esthetician uses professional products that are not available at retail. Therefore, you would not be able to exactly replicate the service at home.

"At home, in between facials, I recommend buying a five-time magnifying mirror with a light. It just gets you to be more meticulous, and after a facial, I can check to make sure everything is out. If it is, the esthetician has me hooked and has made me very happy. After your acne facial, scrub two to three times a week with Botanical Buffing Beads. An acne gel with AHA is also good for blackheads (AHA/BHA Acne Clearing Gel) because the AHA gets in there and gets rid of the black in the blackheads. It helps dissolve the black color so you don't see it, and the BHA controls your acne." Peter Thomas Roth

Squeeze Softly

"In some regards, blackheads are the most stubborn problem. The tendency to have blackheads is more genetically determined than anything else. If you are susceptible to blackheads, any lotions, creams, or oils—even if they are essential oils—will cause this problem. The bottom line is that the primary way to get rid of them is to gently remove them by squeezing. Now, I know squeezing can be damaging to the skin, but it's how you squeeze that determines whether or not it is really damaging for the skin. If you over-squeeze, pinch the skin, scrape the skin with your nails, or press too hard, you absolutely are damaging the skin. Gentle is the operative word, and when done right, squeezing is the best—if not only—way to clean blackheads. Steaming your face can also help remove blackheads, but be careful how long you steam. Five minutes is enough. After steaming, squeeze gently, and splash with cold water to close pores. Do not remove blackheads more than once a week." Giella

THE BENZOYL-PEROXIDE DEBATE

The Buzz from the Beauty Editor

It's easy to dismiss benzoyl peroxide. After all, you probably dabbed it on pimples as a teenager. By now, there's got to be something better, right? Wrong. The truth is, benzoyl peroxide is an extremely potent antibacterial agent, but for years, it was being used incorrectly. Benzoyl peroxide is most effective when it is used regularly, all over the infected area, and not occasionally as a spot treatment. If your skin can tolerate it without excessive irritation, it can be an important element of any acne-fighting routine.

Insider Information from the Beauty Bunch

BP for Breakouts

"The best topical agent that a woman can use for breakouts is benzoyl peroxide. A lot of people don't understand that benzoyl peroxide is the most effective antibacterial agent ever invented. You never develop a resistance to it, so you can use it your whole life. It kills acne bacteria more effectively than anything. You have to use it proactively, for prevention, and not just to spot treat. Here's my recommended regimen: at night, do your regular skin-care program for your skin type, using your anti-aging products. Then, put the benzoyl peroxide on the breakout-prone areas right over the rest of your skin-care products. Choose your benzoyl peroxide product carefully. It has to be a good formulation. Most have a lot of unnecessary ingredients in them.

I have helped a lot of adult women completely clear up their acne using this method alone." Jan Marini

Inflammatory Statements

"If you get control of inflammation, you get control of acne. That's why products that cause irritation should be used in moderation, if at all. Benzoyl peroxide is irritating, for example, but it does kill bacteria. It's a vicious cycle because when your skin is inflamed or irritated, an enzyme called hyaluronidase is released. Hyaluronidase consumes hyaluronic acid, which is one of the primary components of the dermis. With chronic acne, long-term exposure to hyaluronidase ultimately dissolves the matrix at the base of the pore, which is in your dermis, causing the surrounding area to collapse, and leading to scarring and pitting." Gabrielle Ophals

Pimple Prescription

"If you have a huge, painful pimple, you should have a dermatologist take a look at it, and possibly suggest he/she remove it or inject it with cortisol so that it goes away and doesn't scar. A cystic blemish that can't be removed might also cause a scar. What I've also found is that any blemish, small or large, might scar. So the good news is that you can have a whopper of a zit and it doesn't necessarily mean it will scar. When benzoyl peroxide or salicylic acid is used every night, it's very effective, and it starts working immediately. Benzoyl peroxide can bleach your pillowcase, though, so you might want to use a white pillowcase or, if it's too late, flip it over to hide the staining.

"If your skin is sensitive to benzoyl peroxide, and salicylic acid does not work for you, put it on for twenty minutes and then wash it off to build up your tolerance from there. The next day, leave it on for an hour, then two hours the day after that, and so on. Your skin will get used to it and won't dry out, and you'll be able to tolerate it all night long. If you're the type of person who wakes up with two pimples every day, start with five-percent benzoyl peroxide, and if that doesn't work, go up to ten percent and add a sulfur mask. For very light acne, five percent is fine. If you wake up with dry, flaky skin, use a mild scrub or put a mask on for ten minutes and wash it off in the shower. It gets rid of the flakes." Peter Thomas Roth

Going Underground

"I hate when I get those 'undergrounder' pimples—the painful red ones that you can't extract and take forever to resolve. To speed things along, when I'm in the shower, I take a cleansing gel and gently massage it in an upwards fashion with two fingers from the base—try to get underneath it from the sides and very, very gently massage upwards for about thirty seconds. Only once a whitehead appears can you have it successfully extracted by a professional esthetician.

"I also try not to use too many drying or irritating products on it—even though it's difficult to resist—because it's already so inflamed. Plus, the last thing you want to do is dry out the skin on top of and around it. Save the drying potions for after extraction. I also find that a five- to ten-minute mask of a five-percent benzoyl peroxide product under an ice pack once a day can help—but be sure to remove the benzoyl peroxide because it can be very irritating to the skin, and irritation exacerbates acne. The cold compress accelerates the penetration of the product into the skin—when you apply cold to something, it contracts—drawing the product in deeper on its way. In concentrations of two percent and higher, benzoyl peroxide is considered an over-the-counter drug by the FDA, and therefore must be labeled as such. Also, acne bacteria do not build up a resistance to benzoyl peroxide—whereas they do

with pretty much all antibiotics eventually, which is why people with acne find that certain medications just stop working for them after a while." Gabrielle Ophals

ANTI-AGING AGENDA

The Buzz from the Beauty Editor

I've been obsessed with the fight against aging since the tender age of twenty-one. My mother, on the other hand, considers each birthday a blessing, and subsequently, her skin-care routine is of the soap-and-water variety. Somewhere in the middle is a happy medium. Combine the courage to grow old gracefully with some simple, skin-saving anti-aging strategies, and you'll age happily and beautifully.

Insider Information from the Beauty Bunch

Multitasking

"I believe all anti-aging products should combine multiple anti-aging ingredients so that the product/formula has the ability to: combat and protect against free-radical damage; soothe stressed skin to avoid free-radical damage; nourish and strengthen the skin; reduce the visible signs of aging through stimulating collagen production and the growth of healthy young cells—without causing irritation and/or inflammation. When irritation or inflammation is present, free radicals run rampant and this can lead to premature aging. Ideally, the products should contain chirally correct ingredients, since [they] increase the effectiveness of the ingredients while reducing the chance of inflammation/irritation." Shan Albert

Anti-Aging Essentials
"Everyone in my office, male or female, regardless of age, is advised to use sunscreen with zinc oxide in the morning and a retinoid in the evening. The retinoid I choose depends on the skin they have. With acne, it's Retin-A, which kills two birds with one stone. It addresses acne and stimulates collagen. If a patient is in her thirties, then maybe it will be a retinol, which is less irritating. For a more mature woman in her fifties, with dryer skin, I might prescribe Renova, which has mineral oil." Jessica Wu, MD

Peel Appeal
"Home peels are essential, and they're gentle enough to use every day. The pH fluctuation from step one to step two [in MD Skincare's Alpha Beta Daily Face Peel] is a mechanism that allows the skin to produce more collagen and makes existing collagen resort to a more pristine structure." Dennis Gross, MD

Triple Threat
To prevent aging: "Protect the skin from inflammation and keep it calm, because inflammation results in the overproduction of destructive free radicals; protect the skin with antioxidants to keep destructive free radicals under control, and provide the skin with the nourishment it needs." Shan Albert

Four Essential Anti-Agers
"I think that the consumer today should look at product ingredients. There are four categories that help revive and preserve collagen. Collagen is the key structural protein in the skin that gives it firmness. Collagen is to skin what calcium is to bones. When it starts to break down, it will lead to fine lines, wrinkles, and laxity. But we cannot put collagen into a cream and put it onto the skin. It will not penetrate, because it's too large a protein. So we need to boost our skin's ability to produce it, and preserve the existing collagen. You need to look for ingredients that target that one specific protein.

"The first thing you need to do is boost collagen, and the best way to do this is through vitamin C, topically applied. It is more important to apply it than to consume it, because it's more direct. You would have to consume one hundred vitamin-C tablets a day to get the same benefit to your skin as you would in a vitamin-C gel. When you take a vitamin-C tablet, it goes into your bloodstream and goes through your whole body; it's diluted so much. I'm not saying to not take vitamin C. I'm not an opponent of good nutrition or supplementation. I am simply saying that your skin needs it in a more direct form. Other collagen boosters include lasers and soy isoflavones like genestein.

"The second group of ingredients you need to look for are peptides.

"The third group is antioxidants. Antioxidants reduce free radicals, which destroy collagen. There's a different mechanism involved in losing collagen than in losing the ability to produce collagen. Antioxidants all work under different conditions. Use a host of antioxidants. Don't buy a product with just one ingredient in it; you'll be missing out on half a dozen others. That's why I consolidate them. I like products that contain multiactive ingredients. The antioxidants to look for are green tea, vitamin C (which also serves as an antioxidant), coenzyme Q10, emblica (used in ayurvedic medicine), grapeseed extract, selenium, and lycopene. I put all of these in my products, in the same concentrations that you would find in a single-ingredient product.

"And finally, there are enzymes in the skin that break down collagen. Retinol helps block this degradation, so it's the final key ingredient to look for. Genestein also has this effect." Dennis Gross, MD

Anti-Age Regimen

"The most common mistake women make with their skin is to assume that just washing their face once or twice a day and applying a moisturizer is sufficient to 'age gracefully.' An anti-aging regimen is the most important aspect in trying to reverse and prevent aging. For the daily regimen, cleanse every morning and every night, preferably with a gentle foaming cleanser one of those times and a slightly more abrasive but non-irritating cleanser perhaps once every night or every second or third night, depending on skin sensitivity. Sun-screening is essential and should be applied year-round. Then, I recommend a retinoid, and a botanical such as green tea extract or another antioxidant such as vitamin C. Please note that no twelve-hour period should pass without an active ingredient being applied to the face. If sunscreens are used, then a combination sunscreen and anti-aging product is appropriate, or an anti-aging product may be applied under the sunscreen so that during the day, the individual has both sunscreen on and something that is helping to reverse the aging process. At night, of course, after cleansing, at least one anti-aging product should be applied. The regimen described above is essential for all women to maintain the appearance of the skin and to enhance its beauty. The best way to avoid the need for cosmetic surgical procedures is to take care of one's skin from early childhood by avoiding sun, by using sun protection, and [by] having a daily regimen that one sticks to. The most common complaint that my patients have about their skin is that they look older than they feel. [The solution is the regimen described above.]" Jeffrey Dover, MD

Miracle Workers

"I tend to dismiss any ingredient that promises, by itself, to rejuvenate the skin (what I call 'miracle ingredients') because skin aging is multi-factorial. Look, for example, at the news release that claimed a scientist at Clarkson University has discovered why older skin feels 'leathery': the cytoskeleton of epithelial cells becomes more rigid. I have no problem in accepting that the cytoskeleton, the protein net that helps the cell keeps its shape, changes with the skin's age. But what about all the other changes we know happen in skin cells and in the dermis? Collagen and elastin, deep in the dermis, are modified in ways that affect their elasticity, and so the epidermis changes in many other ways in addition to whatever happens to the cytoskeleton. This miracle ingredient won't work for the other factors that make a skin look old. In short, miracle ingredients (the 'one' that will make you young again) work only for marketing." Shan Albert

SPECIFIC CONCERNS

The Buzz from the Beauty Editor

My magnifying mirror is one of my most prized possessions, and over the years, it's shown me the error of my ways. From clogged pores to dry patches, I've seen all too clearly when my current skin-care strategies are not working. Recently, it pointed out that a tiny little white bump under my eye was actually a milium, and not a whitehead, and that the freckle on my upper lip meant I needed to better protect this fragile area with sunscreen. If your skin-care issues include milia and rosacea, read on for some potential treatments.

Insider Information from the Beauty Bunch

Wiping Out White Bumps

"Many women suffer from small, white, hard bumps on their cheeks and undereye area. These bumps are probably milia, and they are painful. Milia are tiny sebum-filled cysts near the surface of the skin. Though these cysts generally occur in those with oily, acne-prone skin, they occasionally show up on women with dry skin. The probable cause is the buildup of greasy moisturizers or cleansers that are too emollient and contain pore-clogging ingredients. Wearing glasses can also cause a ridge of white bumps where the frame contacts the skin. The rubbing stimulates the oil glands, creating the cysts. These bumps aren't easy to remove on your own, especially if they are by your eyes. An ophthalmologist or dermatologist can remove them. To avoid having the bumps return, find a pair of glasses that do not rest on the face and eliminate heavy, thick moisturizers and cleansers." Giella

Rosacea Rundown

"Rosacea is a very common condition in America consisting of redness, flushing, telangiectasia [dilated blood vessels], and red papules and pustules. It is usually very easy to recognize. There is no cure. Avoid irritating and precipitating factors such as heat, hot foods, spicy foods, and other causes of flushing. Treatment includes both topical treatments like Metronidazole and sometimes topical antibiotics, systemic antibiotics, and laser or light treatment for the redness, the flushing, and the telangiectasia." Jeffrey Dover, MD

Rosacea Red Light

"Rosacea is progressive, affects far more women than men, and is much more frequent in fairer skin. The onset is usually between the ages of thirty and fifty. It is unlikely, but the onset can occur in adolescents and the elderly. No one knows what causes rosacea, but one of the primary causative factors is cumulative sun exposure." Jan Marini

HALTING HYPERPIGMENTATION

The Buzz from the Beauty Editor

With my olive skin, hyperpigmentation is always a risk. Hyperpigmentation is a condition in which the skin produces too much melanin, the brown pigment that gives your skin its color. This leads to brown spots, freckles, and dark patches. I try to prevent picking, poking, or irritating it in any way, since this inevitably leads to dark spots. I also use my sunscreen religiously, since sun exposure tends to bring out the brown. And finally, I treat it with specifically designed fading creams.

Insider Information from the Beauty Bunch

Types of Hyperpigmentation

"There are a variety of causes of hyperpigmentation. There is sun-induced dyspigmentation with lentigines [sun spots] and freckles. This can be prevented with sun avoidance and sunscreen, but does not respond to topical lightening agents in spite of the fact that they are used extensively for this. The only effective treatments are lasers and light treatments. All the Q-switched lasers and intense pulsed light sources are effective when used properly by experts to treat this condition. The other common causes of hyperpigmentation are melasma and post-inflammatory hyperpigmentation. These do not typically respond to laser treatment, but do respond to sun avoidance and skin-lightening agents including four-percent hydroquinone, which we like to use in combination with retinoids and topical steroids. These are prescription items not available over-the-counter. There are over-the-counter lightening agents with two-percent hydroquinone and other lightening agents available over the counter which individuals can try before seeing a dermatologist for this problem. Occasionally, they do not need the prescription concentration." Jeffrey Dover, MD

Best Brighteners

"Magnesium ascorbyl phosphate is the number-one skin brightener in Japan. It is safe and a good antioxidant, too. In the U.S., hydroquinone and kojic acid are popular, but retinoids also have a place." Mary Lupo, MD

White Spot Warning

"Azelaic acid—Azelex—gets rid of acne marks faster when used in small percentages. But be careful. In high percentages, it can leave little white spots, hypopigment, because it's a pigment-lifting agent." Jan Marini

Lighten Up

"Hydroquinone is a powerful skin lightener, and you have to be careful with it. It can actually cause the skin to lose pigment and become lighter than the skin around it. Also, you can't use it for a long time because it affects your liver. That's why it's only available through a doctor. Over-the-counter products tend to be less aggressive than the prescription ones. I like SkinCeuticals Phyto +. You apply it underneath your moisturizer, and it uses natural ingredients like kojic acid to just even out skintone. It only works if the brown spots are sun-induced; if they are hormone-induced, you'll need hydroquinone." Gabrielle Ophals

Brown-Spot Banisher

"Intense Pulsed Light, IPL, is one option for eliminating brown spots. For Asian and Hispanic patients, combine IPL with chemical peels. All my patients are on a homecare routine to prep skin before, during, and after their series of treatments, and the routine includes sunscreen as well as a prescription-strength fading cream, which usually contains hydroquinone. It depends on the depth of the pigment. Some acne scars are dark red, not brown, so fading creams won't do anything for them, and maybe IPL is better. Kojic acid is not as strong as hydroquinone, but some people are sensitive or don't want to use hydroquinone for some reason, so kojic acid is an alternative." Jessica Wu, MD

INGREDIENT ANALYSIS

The Buzz from the Beauty Editor

Skin-care ingredients can be baffling, even for those of us who make it our business to keep up with this stuff. New "miracle" discoveries are made almost daily, and to further complicate the matter, it's not only the presence of an ingredient, but the concentration and composition of a product that makes it either effective or virtually useless. When I'm in doubt, I turn to a dermatologist or ingredient expert to help me decipher the labels, as I've done in this section.

Insider Information from the Beauty Bunch

Effective Concentration

"Anti-aging ingredients need to be present in the product in a high enough concentration (or percentage) to be effective. Additionally they should be in a 'safe' base—one with ingredients that allow the skin to function properly. This means the base should be water-soluble, not occlusive. Examples of bases that are occlusive are those that contain petrolatum or even natural waxes. Natural products should also be free of artificial colors, artificial fragrances, and ideally artificial preservatives (such as parabens). It is the combination of ingredients in a formula that makes all the difference, not just one or two special ingredients." Shan Albert

Correct Composition of Ingredients

"There are a lot of good ingredients, but the key is how they are used. It's not just the presence of the ingredient that makes the product effective, but the base, or vehicle. Water, emulsifiers, and preservatives are all parts of the vehicle that carry the performance ingredients. [In skin care, the correct term is performance ingredients, not active ingredients, the correct term for drugs.]

"Ingredients have to be listed in descending order of predominance. The ingredients that amount to less than one percent of the product can be listed in any order the manufacturer wants. Some performance ingredients are good in low quantities and oth-

ers are good in high quantities. Hyaluronic acid, for example, is very moisturizing, but you want to see it at the middle of the ingredient list, or about one percent of the product. On most ingredient labels, if you have ten ingredients, then you'll find the products that compose one percent of the product about halfway down the label. The more ingredients you get, the higher one percent will be on the list, maybe within the first five to seven ingredients. Ingredients that fall after preservatives, of which parabens are the most common, are probably less than half a percent of the product. In skin care, ingredients that come after fragrance are also less than half a percent. Ingredients that come after fragrance in a body-care product can be about three to five percent of the product, because body products contain much more fragrance." Rebecca James Gadberry

Taut Jaw

"Acetylcholine is not the whole answer to the aging process, but [it is] a piece of it. A precursor to acetylcholine, also known as a 'neuro-transmitter' factor, is in every single [Jan Marini Skin Research] C-Esta product. Every cell in your body has a receptor site for acetylcholine, and among other things, it plays a role in correct anatomical muscle positioning. Muscle elongation happens throughout the body, including the face. The facial nerve sparks acetylcholine into the muscle and causes the muscle to shorten, which assists in maintaining well-defined facial contours. By enhancing acetylcholine, you see immediate short-term benefits in two to three minutes and longer-term progressive benefits, and these benefits, over a period of time, become permanent. Johnson & Johnson did a double-blind study at the University of Pennsylvania and saw significant improvement in skin texture, jowls, sagging, droopiness of the eyebrows, and crepeyness of the eyelids." Jan Marini

Finding Gentle AHAs

"The problem with AHAs is that they are very irritating. I could not use glycolic acids until the amphoteric AHAs came out. To address the problem, doctors Eugene Van Scott and Ruey Yu, who invented AHAs, simply linked molecules together to make a larger molecule, which slows down penetration. The problem is that it wasn't as effective. Now they've attached a pilot molecule, an amino acid named arginine, which stabilizes the AHA in the product and carries it into the skin so that there is a time release. Instead of getting peak delivery in one and a half to three minutes, it takes seven to fifteen minutes. This reduces the stinging, but the same amount is delivered. It's slower delivery but total delivery. To find an amphoteric AHA, look for lactic acid and glycolic acid first, and then arginine lower on the ingredient list." Rebecca James Gadberry

Why Water Could Be Damaging Your Skin

"There's a residue in water that can have negative effects on skin. Tap water contains heavy metals, like iron, magnesium, zinc, copper, and lead, that are free radicals, and by washing your face in them you're doing damage. I've developed an ingredient called Hydrapure to solve this problem. It has a chelating complex, like little Pac Men, that engulfs and encapsulates the free radicals. It can actually reverse these heavy metals and stop yet another source of free radicals. It really is an innovation. It all goes back to the main goal of building and preserving collagen. To really get the best skin you have to make sure nature's mechanisms work better. If water is not pure, it will be a problem; if you can improve the water, you've turned a big negative into a tremendous positive. Also, calcium and magnesium can cause one's own oils to become comedogenic. Heavy metals and calcium together can cause breakouts. I have patients who travel all over the world, including beauty edi-

tors who were returning from Fashion Week in Milan, with irritation, breakouts, rashes, and rosacea. Once I gave them the chelating product, they had no problem the next time. They couldn't believe it was the water they were washing their faces with that caused breakouts." Dennis Gross, MD

Firming Find

"There's a new protein that a lot of companies are using that is a topical firming protein. It comes from sweet almond seed extract. It forms a three-dimensional matrix on the skin, like an invisible network that attaches to points between your skin cells. This causes an immediate firming and lifting of the skin. It's an amazing ingredient that comes out of France. It's a protein, not a peptide. It creates anchors between the cells, but it doesn't penetrate. It's being used for the face, to lift eyes, neck, and facial contours, and for the body, in cellulite products." Rebecca James Gadberry

An AHA Lesson

"AHAs are alpha hydroxy acids, and they are the big umbrella group of fruit acids. There are many different types of fruit acids, such as glycolic acid, the most popular, made from sugar cane; malic acid made from apples; citric acid made from lemon and limes; lactic acid made from sour milk; and kojic acid made from mushrooms.

"Glycolic acid, being the most popular, is recommended by many dermatologists and has many benefits. It improves skin texture and pigmentation problems, controls excessive oiliness, unclogs pores, and minimizes ingrown hairs. Most dermatologists will recommend an AHA for controlling acne or for treating fine lines and wrinkles. It is recommended that the glycolic acid be ten percent or higher—anything less is not effective. Ask the percentage of glycolic acid in a particular cream before you buy it.

If it is unknown, avoid it. It is also helpful to know the pH level, which tells how active the ingredient is in the cream. Seven is the lowest and one is the highest. The GIELLA Renouveau contains a ten-percent glycolic acid with a pH of a three-point-eight percent.

"You can use Retin-A and glycolic acid together. For instance, you can alternate using Retin-A one night and glycolic acid another night, or you can use Retin-A at night and glycolic acid in the morning. If you do use them together, apply the Retin-A first, and then the glycolic acid cream over it. Always use sunscreen when using both Retin-A and glycolic acid—at least an SPF fifteen or higher." Giella

The Cosmetic Question

"Cosmetics do not permanently affect the skin. We can only provide temporary relief and changes. The idea is to use them regularly. Some ingredients do have a cumulative effect; like sweet almond seed extract. If it isn't covered by a drug monograph [the regulatory standards for marketing a drug], then you cannot make the claim that it affects the dermis of the skin. The FDA draws the line at the stratum corneum. Any claims made for products below the stratum corneum are considered drug claims. If you say a product works in the dermis, you're making a drug claim.

"There are no monographs for anti-aging. If you make an anti-aging claim, you need FDA clearance, unless you use helper words (seems to, appears, et cetera). For example, if I want to make the claim that a product will permanently eliminate wrinkles around the eyes, I need to do a lot of research, spend millions of dollars, and make a claim for it as a drug, which could take many years. The claim needs to be made for the product, not the ingredient. If a product does work in the dermis, but you don't make that claim, then it's okay. It's the intent for the product at point of sale, rather than what the product actually does, that determines whether the FDA will step in.

"This is the problem faced by the cosmetic industry. There are a number of ingredients that work really well, but we're not allowed to say anything about them. A lot of dermatologists say that cosmetics don't work because they don't affect the stratum corneum, and by definition that is true, but in reality it's a different situation. The ingredient may work on that level, but the company cannot make that claim." Rebecca James Gadberry

EGF Excitement

"The nearest we get to a miracle ingredient is epidermal growth factor, which is derived from yeast. EGF is a serum protein whose binding to a specific receptor on the cell surface initiates a cascade of molecular events that will lead, among other effects, to cell division. EGF accelerates healing of the skin and the cornea. It has been demonstrated that EGF can stimulate dermal repair. EGF supplied to the skin increases mitosis, synthesis of proteins, the number of fibroblasts, the accumulation of collagen, circulation, and mediation of blood-vessel formulation." Shan Albert

Why You Need Vitamin C

"Your skin is exposed to environmental elements such as sunlight and air pollution every day. These elements cause free radicals to form in the skin, which attack the skin's collagen layer. This process prematurely ages and damages the skin, resulting in fine lines and wrinkles, loss of elasticity, and hyperpigmentation. This process is known as photo-aging. Vitamin-C products provide antioxidant protection from environmental damage. However, it is important to use products that contain at least eight- to ten-percent vitamin C. Continued use of vitamin-C products may improve the overall health and appearance of your skin." Giella

The Retinoid Breakdown

"Retinoids are in the vitamin-A family. Look for 'retin' in the name. The reason that vitamin A works in the skin is that all cells except red blood cells have vitamin-A receptors. Vitamin A is part of what tells the cells to go into mitosis, to split apart and form new cells. It's a messenger molecule for cells in your skin.

"Retinol is the alcohol form of vitamin A. Retinoic acid is the most active form of vitamin A. Retinol palmitate and beta carotene are the storage forms of vitamin A. Your skin turns them into the active form of retinol when it needs it. You can have them on your skin, but if your cells don't need it, it won't turn it into vitamin A. A receptor on a cell is like the lock on the front door of your house; the lock is the mirror image of the key you use to open it. The receptor is the mirror image of the molecule that it is going to receive, or the mirror pattern. When the retinol goes into the cell, the cell turns it into retinol aldehyde, which becomes retinoic acid.

"All forms of vitamin A have activity of some sort. Weaker retinols are less effective, but less likely to irritate. Retinol palmitate is the mildest and weakest. Retinol is stronger and more likely to irritate. Retinal aldehyde and retinoic acid are the most likely to irritate, but have the most activity. Retinol has one-tenth the activity of retinoic acid (i.e., Retin-A, Renova). Retinol can be a skin lightener, it can fight wrinkles by boosting collagen, and it can help skin slough off the old barrier to soften skin. You want to see retinol towards the bottom of label." Rebecca James Gadberry

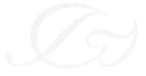

THE PEPTIDE CHALLENGE

The Buzz from the Beauty Editor

I am always the first to incorporate the hottest, newest skin-care ingredients into my routine, so when peptides popped up, I rushed out to buy a peptide cream. I have found it to be a useful addition to my skin-care routine, but like any other single ingredient, peptides alone won't work miracles. Even though they are shaping up to be the breakthrough of the decade, in much the same way that alpha hydroxy acids revolutionized skin-care in the last decade, their ultimate effectiveness has yet to be determined. Read on to see whether peptides deserve a place in your skin-care routine.

Insider Information from the Beauty Bunch

Problem with Peptides

"There are some peptides that are very interesting. They are good for people who can't tolerate retinoids, but there's clearly much more data on retinoids. But not everyone can tolerate them. Peptides are a good alternative for people who can't use retinoids at all, or who can only use them a couple of times a week. On in-between nights, use peptides." Jessica Wu, MD

The Next Big Thing

"Peptides are the new big thing in skin care, replacing AHAs, vitamin C, and retinol. They are being used primarily in anti-aging products, but also in some anti-acne products. They are easier to work with, easier to put into a product, less irritating or not irritating at all, and they are more compatible with a number of other ingredients.

"Peptides are fragments of proteins that are frequently used as signal messengers, signaling molecules to make dermal tissue to fill out the mattress underneath your skin. It plumps up the dermal tissue, which plumps up the lines above so that they fill out. It acts sort of like Restylane or some of those other line fillers out there. It is the next wave of high-performance skin-care ingredients, and ingredient suppliers are putting a lot of money right now into researching different types of peptides. Peptides are smaller than proteins, and have a higher affinity for the skin. They seem to work better when they have a pilot molecule attached to them, usually a fatty molecule. The fatty molecules carry the peptide into the skin and then release it. So, when looking at an ingredient list, you should find one of these pilot molecules—palmitoyl, oleyl, acetyl, or myristyl—in the peptide name. Look for peptides anywhere from the second ingredient to halfway down the ingredient list."

Skin-Care Issue
Undereye circles
Proper Peptide
Look for palmitoyl oligopeptide together with palmitoyl tetrapeptide-3.

Skin-Care Issue
Botox alternative
Proper Peptide
Look for dipeptide-2 and palmitoyl tetrapeptide-3.

Skin-Care Issue
Fuller lips, fresher eyes

Proper Peptide
Hydrolyzed hibiscus esculentus extract, which comes from okra, works on the surface of the skin, sort of like Botox.

Skin-Care Issue
Firmness, elasticity
Proper Peptide
Dipeptide-2 can reduce puffiness around the eye, plump up lips, and reduce undereye circles.

Skin-Care Issue
Fill in fine lines
Proper Peptide
Pisum sativum extract, which comes from peas, neutralizes enzymes that destroy the elastin and collagen in the skin. It's an anti-enzyme that stimulates elastin so that the skin is firmer.

Combine pisum sativum with bambusa vulgaris (bamboo) extract to boost collagen and dermal tissue. It functions sort of like Restylane.

Rebecca James Gadberry

The Peptide Prescription
"Peptides, growth factors, et cetera, may have a place [in skin care], but absorption issues must be addressed." Mary Lupo, MD

Points for Peptides
"Peptides are a new class of anti-aging drugs which I think make a nice addition to a skin-care regimen, [but] which should not be the base of the regimen." Jeffrey Dover, MD

ANALYZING ANTIOXIDANTS

The Buzz from the Beauty Editor

Antioxidants are an essential element of any skin-care routine, and new ones are being discovered all the time. The latest crop of antioxidants are derived from nature: cranberries, green tea, grapeseeds. Whether the source is synthetic or natural, all antioxidants function in much the same manner: they protect the skin from destructive free radicals.

Insider Information from the Beauty Bunch

How Antioxidants Work

"Antioxidants work by blocking and interrupting the oxygen metabolic pathway in the skin. UV exposure to skin converts oxygen O_2 into singlet oxygen O_1, which is very inflammatory and causes destruction of cells through an inflammatory free radical metabolic pathway. By quenching these free radicals, one can decrease the ill effects of the sun on the skin, which is why we like topical vitamins C and E, antioxidants, grapeseed extract, and a variety of other botanicals including green tea and black tea." Jeffrey Dover, MD

Antioxidant Answers

"Antioxidants are not always stable; they do react with oxygen. If you expose them to sunlight or oxygen, they oxidize and turn brown. After turning brown they will no longer be protective and will be an irritant. A lot of people think that vitamin C clogs pores, but it only does so if it's oxidized. Vitamin C (sodium ascorbyl phosphate) and vitamin E (toco-pheryl acetate) in really low quantities combined with a sunscreen help reduce the amount of free radicals on the skin caused by sunlight. 'Tocoph' indicates vitamin E, and 'ascorb' indicates some form of vitamin C." Rebecca James Gadberry

Antioxidant Analysis

"The skin is composed of an oil phase and a lipid phase. The membranes of the skin are composed of lipids, and inside the cells are phytoplasms, or liquid. Some antioxidants are water-soluble and some are lipid-soluble. [The] consumer should use antioxidants that are both water-soluble and lipid-soluble, like vitamin C. You need to get to both segments of the skin." Dennis Gross, MD

Wine Country

"Grapeseed extract is one of the most effective antioxidant ingredients in skin care. It provides more antioxidant power than vitamins C, E, and beta carotene. It also has the ability to bind to collagen and thereby promotes youthful skin, healthy cells, cellular elasticity, and flexibility. The best grapeseed extract is derived from an all-natural cold filter process. It is not extracted with the use of chemicals. This results in a finer extract that absorbs more easily. " Jim Miller

Antioxidants Aplenty

"It is important to use more than one antioxidant in a formulation because reactive oxygen species attack our lipids, membrane structures, and our bodies at a multitude of points. It is impossible to tell exactly where a particular antioxidant will act, and it will probably work at many different points. We gain from using several different antioxidants because we increase the chances of having effective antioxidants at crucial attack points." Shan Albert

Prevage Perspective

"There is a lot of media hype about Prevage because it's new, but the study has not been published yet. Most of us in the medical community are waiting for the results before we comment on it. Potentially, it sounds like an amazing antioxidant, and it appears to be stronger than anything else out there, but the only materials we have to go by are what the company has released. Everyone's clamoring for it, but most doctors tend to be a little more conservative. We wait until we see the research. We want to make sure patients are happy." Jessica Wu, MD

Cranberry Connection

"One very good source of vitamin E is cranberry oil, which has all eight forms of vitamin E in it. It's very unique. It acts as a natural total antioxidant for the skin. Vitamin E helps to keep the stratum corneum moist and flexible, so skin is really soft. There should be about one percent of it in a product; look for it in the second half of an ingredient list." Rebecca James Gadberry

THE PRODUCT FILES

Masks

The Buzz from the Beauty Editor

I get a professional facial every four weeks, but for between-facial maintenance, nothing beats a good mask. I've always reached for clay masks to treat my combination, pimple-prone skin, but as I get older, I've branched out and discovered that hydrating masks can also have a beneficial effect. Masks should not be rubbed in like moisturizer. They should be applied liberally, spread onto the surface of the skin (no rubbing or massaging in), and left to dry according to the instructions on the package. My favorites are Face Stockholm Sage & Aloe Mask, $18, and Awake Vital Express Mask, $55.

What the Pros Choose

Many pros seem to want some muscle in their masks, choosing hardworking formulas like Haven Porification Mask (Gabrielle Ophals), Bliss Sleeping Peel Microexfoliating Mask (Wende Zomnir), Aveda Tourmaline Charged Radiance Mask (Shauna Raisch), Catherine Atzen Biological Modeling Mask (Vanessa Talabac), Daniello Instant Beauty Mask (Lilly Rivera), and Sircuit Skin Cosmeceuticals Sir-Activ Zeolite Purifying Scrub (Shan Albert). Others go for moisturizing formulas, like Prada Hydrating Mask (Meg Thompson) and Boscia Moisture Replenishing Lotion (Meredith Green, who uses it as a mask), or skin-boosting ones, like Clarins Beauty Flash Balm (Julie Hewett). Still others turn to nature for inspiration, as in Enessa Replenishing Moor Mask (Michelle Ornstein); to the sea, as in Avancé Purifying Sea Mask (Dee DeLuca-Mattos); and to fruits and vegetables, as in Peter Thomas Roth Cucumber Gel Masque (Peter Thomas Roth), and June Jacobs Pumpkin Masque and Cranberry Pomegranate Masque (June Jacobs).

Acne Treatments

The Buzz from the Beauty Editor

Having struggled with persistent breakouts for years, I've tried almost every acne treatment on the market. I know what works, and what does more harm than good. And I've also learned that consistency is the key to great skin—give a product three months before determining whether or not it's working. If you're looking to prevent acne, good old benzoyl peroxide works miracles. The key is to apply it regularly, and use it all over acne-prone areas. If a spot treatment is what you're looking for, nothing beats salicylic acid. My favorites are Jan Marini Benzoyl Peroxide 5% Lotion, $21, and Neutrogena Clear Pore Treatment, $8.

What the Pros Choose

Familiar favorites appear on this list alongside some cult classics. Clearasil is the treatment of choice for Wende Zomnir and Meredith Green. Spaworthy picks include the acne-skin-care line from Kinara Spa (Julie Hewett), Avancé Algae Deep Gentle Cleanse (Dee DeLuca-Mattos), Catherine Atzen AM-PM Purifying Gel (Vanessa Talabac), Aveda Balancing Infusion for Oily Skin/Acne (Shauna Raisch), and Enessa Clove Oil (Michelle Ornstein). Peter Thomas Roth and June Jacobs both choose Roth's own formulas; Jacobs specifies his AHA/BHA Acne Clearing Gel. Other picks include Proactiv Solution (Mala Elhassan), Mario Badescu Drying Lotion (Hara Glick), and The Vital Image Acneno (Linda Deslauriers). Shan Albert chooses Cosmedix Clear Medical Clarifier because it's "chirally correct, meaning that it provides the finest results with the fewest possible side effects." Danielle Browning has the most unusual pick: she chooses facials, rather than an individual product, as the best acne treatment. Gabrielle Ophals picks Yon-Ka Crème 11: "I like that Yon-Ka's philosophy is that problem skin needs to be treated as gently as possible, and that the primary goal is to reduce irritation. The Crème 11 is known in our spa as Cream '911' for its ability to bring down inflammation."

Anti-Aging Treatments

The Buzz from the Beauty Editor

I've recently admitted, much to my dismay, that it's time I got serious about anti-aging skin care. Fortunately, I've been using eye creams and sunscreen for years, but now that my skin is slightly less oily than it was in my youth, I am feeling the need for products designed to address more than just breakouts. I need something that will treat signs of aging—fine lines, hyperpigmentation, dullness—without clogging pores or exacerbating my troubled skin. If you suffer from adult acne and early signs of aging, like me, look for an anti-aging product in lotion, serum, or gel form, as opposed to a cream. Creams can be occlusive, clogging pores and leaving skin greasy. My favorite anti-agers are Neutrogena Healthy Skin Anti-Wrinkle Anti-Blemish Cream, $12, and Z. Bigatti Re-Storation Vitamin and Antioxidant Skin Treatment, $155.

What the Pros Choose

Kinerase shows up on two of the experts' lists (Julie Hewett and Meredith Green), but the rest of the picks range from Botox (Kathryn Alice) to Bliss (Wende Zomnir picks the Bliss Sleeping Peel Serum). Peter Thomas Roth narrows his line down to the Anti-Aging Cleansing Gel and the Power Rescue Facial Firming Lift, while June Jacobs picks her Age Defying Night Complex. Other picks include Avancé Age Defyer (Dee DeLuca-Mattos), MD Formulations

(Mala Elhassan), The Vital Image Lift & Firm Complex and Collagen Builder (Linda Deslauriers), Valmont 24 Hour Cellular Conditioning Base Cream (Danielle Browning), Catherine Atzen Serum Vita C (Vanessa Talabac), Skingenious 10 Years Younger (Shan Albert), and the Pevonia Optimal line (Shauna Raisch).

AHA/Antioxidant Face Products and Serums

The Buzz from the Beauty Editor

Multi-purpose serums, creams, and lotions are the low-maintenance girl's dream: they pack all the benefits of modern skin care into one simple step. Most skin types benefit from one or both of the ingredients in this category: exfoliating, renewing AHAs, and protective, skin-supporting antioxidants. I prefer to use an antioxidant product during the day, when it can best protect my skin from the environment, and an AHA at night, when it can do its work without causing photosensitivity. Acids can be confusing, so here's a little cheat sheet: alpha hydroxy acid, or AHA, is best for aging (A=Aging). AHAs include lactic, glycolic, and citric acids—any of the food-derived acids (lactic acid comes from milk; glycolic, from sugar; and citric, from citrus). BHA, or beta hydroxy acid, is best for breakouts (B=Breakout). Beta hydroxy acid is the same thing as salicylic acid. My favorite antioxidant product is Jan Marini C-Esta Serum/Oil Control, $75, and my favorite AHA is Alpha Hydrox Oil-Free Formula, $10.89.

What the Pros Choose

Since this category is broad, the choices are varied. Picks include Kinara Serum (Julie Hewett), June Jacobs Raspberry Recovery Serum (June Jacobs), Peter Thomas Roth products (Peter Thomas Roth), Avancé Cerum Vitamin C Therapy (Dee DeLuca-Mattos), Catherine Atzen Integral DNA Serum (Vanessa Talabac), Sonya Dakar Omega 3 Repair Complex (Danielle Browning), Boscia Antioxidant Recovery C Treatment (Meredith Green), SkinCeuticals C E Ferulic (Gabrielle Ophals), The Vital Image C-Serum (Linda Deslauriers), Aveda Brightening Essence (Shauna Raisch), and Cosmedix Refine Vitamin A Serum (Shan Albert).

Mattifiers

The Buzz from the Beauty Editor

I live in Florida, where the heat and humidity pose a constant challenge to my oily skin. A mattifier is a daily essential. Without it, skin gets shiny and makeup goes slip-sliding away. Papers and potions both play a role in keeping shine at bay. Apply a mattifying lotion under your makeup, first thing in the morning, to keep skin fresh and matte. If oil begins to break through, use blotting papers to quickly soak up sebum. I prefer powder-free papers, because powdery sheets can make your makeup cakey or cause it to change color. My favorite mattifiers are Origins Zero Oil, $10, and Boscia Fresh Blotting Linens, $6.

What the Pros Choose

From blotting papers to shine-erasing potions, our pros have definite ideas about what it takes to stay matte. On the side of blotting papers, there is Wende

Zomnir with MAC Blotting Film, and Meredith Green with Boscia Blotting Linens. On the lotion side, there's Julie Hewett with Chanel T-Mat Shine Control and Shan Albert with Colorescience Invisibly Matte. Peter Thomas Roth MAX Anti-Shine Mattifying Gel was the pick of Peter Thomas Roth and June Jacobs.

Chapter Three

About Face:
Building the Perfect Base for a Flawless Face

Face makeup is, essentially, non-makeup. When chosen and applied properly, you shouldn't be able to tell it's there. This also makes it the hardest makeup to apply successfully. Foundation is particularly difficult to use, and even trickier to choose. The vast selection of formulas and colors available today makes the process daunting for even the most stalwart beauty addict, but it also increases the likelihood that your perfect fit exists. This chapter will help you zero in on the shades that are most likely to work for you, and shows how you can try before you buy. If you pick your products carefully, foundation should disappear into your skin, highlighter should give you a "natural" glow, blush should make you look healthy and youthful, and bronzer should make you look as though you just returned from vacation—rested and sun-kissed, not orange or muddy.

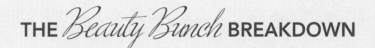

THE *Beauty Bunch* BREAKDOWN

Stephen Sollitto: sought-after celebrity makeup artist whose clients include Christina Aguilera, Rosario Dawson, Jewel, Erika Christensen, and Tara Reid.

Napoleon Perdis: Australian celebrity makeup artist with an eponymous makeup line.

Diane Gardner: Hollywood hairstylist, colorist, and makeup artist, known as the Makeover Specialist.

Kari Boatner: permanent-cosmetics pioneer who has developed innovative instruments and artistic procedures for the application of permanent makeup.

Terri Apanasewicz: celebrity makeup artist with L.A.'s Cloutier Agency whose clients have included Michael Michele, Jeri Ryan, Kristin Davis, Toni Braxton, and Reba McEntire.

Hara Glick: founder of MakeUpAlley.com, the leading consumer beauty product review website.

Meg Thompson: Hollywood makeup artist and co-owner and founder of Madge Cosmetics.

Peter Lamas: founder and chairman of Lamas Beauty International, a rapidly growing, well-respected natural-beauty-product manufacturer.

Galit Strugano: makeup artist and creator of Girlactik Beauty, a topselling makeup line.

Giella: professional makeup artist and founder of GIELLA Custom Blend Cosmetics.

Debra Macki: a top Boston-based makeup artist and the founder of Debra Macki Cosmetics.

Diane Ranger: the founder of mineral makeup and the founder/owner of Colorescience Cosmetics.

Lilly Rivera: celebrated makeup artist at the prestigious Dominique Salon in the Hotel Pierre, New York City.

Wende Zomnir: creative director of Hard Candy Cosmetics and founder/creative director of Urban Decay Cosmetics.

Bobbe Joy: celebrity makeup artist whose clients include Lucy Liu, Scarlett Johansson, Naomi Watts, Jennifer Tilly, and Janice Dickinson, she also has a signature line of products, Makeup! Bobbe Joy.

Mala Elhassan: multitasking miracle-worker who triples as a stylist, colorist, and makeup artist at New York City's hip Robert Kree salon.

Dee DeLuca-Mattos: vice president of Avancé Skincare.

THE BIG PICTURE

The Buzz from the Beauty Editor

Remember when makeup used to be fun? When we first discovered makeup, the urge was to play up our femininity, not to downplay any perceived "flaws." Not knowing what would work for us, we tried everything. As we got older, we lost this sense of possibility and exploration. We now stick with the basics. And soon, our look becomes dated. Trends change rapidly, and last season's dewy look may soon be replaced by a more polished, semi-matte face. Browse fashion magazines and beauty websites occasionally to get a sense of what's current, and don't be afraid to experiment. Don't be a slave to trends, but don't dismiss them either. Try products, formulas, and colors you've never tried before, and then incorporate only what works into your existing makeup routine. To avoid overdoing it, incorporate only one new trend into your existing makeup repertoire at a time.

Insider Information from the Beauty Bunch

Fear Factor

"One of the biggest mistakes that women make with their makeup is being intimidated by it. They make a mistake and never try it again. If they make a mistake with their baby or their boyfriend, they work it through, but if they curl their lashes once and hate it, they never try it again. Don't be afraid of makeup. If you make a mistake, just wash it off. Many women also apply too much color at one time, and end up thinking that the color is wrong for them, when in reality the color is right but the application was heavy. How about a little color at a time? Just try it. For a little color on your lips, take the lipstick and mix it with lip balm for a sheerer application. Wipe off the excess bright blush so it's not so heavy. Same thing with the eyes; a little goes a long way. If you're tentative to try anything creative, start just around your lash line. Anything that you apply just there will not be heavy-handed. As with anything else, you have to persevere if you want to get better." Stephen Sollitto

Rut Reaction

"Women do not change their makeup often enough and get stuck in a rut," says Napoleon Perdis. Diane Gardner agrees: "The one mistake that is consistent with almost every person I see is dated makeup. Women use makeup and techniques from about ten years ago, or when they were first introduced to makeup, and they are stuck in a regimen that no longer suits their features and skin type."

Too Much of a Good Thing

Three pros spoke out against heavy-handed makeup application. According to Kari Boatner, the biggest makeup mistake is "overdoing it. We all have features that are naturally beautiful, but if we wear too much makeup, it causes people to notice the makeup and not the feature." Terri Apanasewicz concurs, saying that the biggest makeup mistake is "too much of it. Women hide behind makeup instead of enhancing their own unique beauty." Hara Glick sums it up: "Don't overdo your makeup. When in doubt, less is more."

Matching Makeup

"I never think about matching the outfit unless it's for a movie, and then I need to know what the actor is wearing. Unless you are talking about wearing bright makeup, your focus should be on choosing colors that look good on you, and on altering your makeup to where you are going. Are you wearing that sundress to church or to a picnic? Adjust your makeup accordingly. Pick what looks best on you and for the occasion. But it's not weird to match lipstick to clothes, especially if you are going for a look. Use your judgment. If you are going for a springtime look and you're wearing pink and green and a babydoll-pink gloss looks beautiful, go for it. But for most women, a natural everyday look that looks best on them is the way to go." Meg Thompson

The Price of Beauty

"With makeup, you pretty much get what you pay for. If you want to look cheap, there's plenty of cheap makeup out there that can help you to achieve that goal. If you want to take good care of your skin, buy a foundation which is natural and healing—and that's probably not going to be cheap." Peter Lamas

Tool Time

Napoleon Perdis considers these three tools indispensable: "A foundation brush, a lip brush to make color even and last longer, and a very wide, flat powder brush, like Perdis's Boudoir brush, which allows powder to be molded with the skin."

PM Perfection

"When you go out at night, you have to add some extra touches to your makeup because the lighting is so dim. I like to do my evening makeup in a dimly lit bathroom so that I can see what it will look like in that light." Meg Thompson

Neutral Territory

"Cosmetic companies know the general behavior of the public, so they sell colors that are not flattering to people. For example, they know that neutrals are safe and they sell a lot of them; ninety-nine percent of women wear all-brown makeup. I see a lot of people's makeup bags, and their makeup is usually beiges, sands, and browns, with the exception of that purple lipstick from ten years ago. The women with vibrant colors are usually artists and creative types.

"I tell my clients that they are picking neutrals because they are safe. And I show them the proper placement of brighter colors. I'll use a teal eye shadow, a bright-peach blush, and a pure-red lip gloss with gold sparkle. Color, color, color. Once they see colors on their face put in the proper place, colors that complement their face, they go out and buy them." Diane Gardner

Looks Can Be Deceiving

"A lot of makeup, particularly blush, looks so different on than in the package. And it wears differently on your skin. That's why you have to try everything on before you buy it. The women at the makeup counters can be helpful because they know whether the colors look the same in the container as they do on your skin, and they know what their top sellers are. When you're applying your makeup, don't worry if you make a mistake. Just fix it or remove it. This happens all the time on a set. You think that something is going to look beautiful on, and then you apply it and it looks awful. You just add more and fix it and keep adjusting until it's right. We blend a million colors together; it's never just one color. You can't say I used that lipstick on her or this eye shadow. And then, for touch-ups, we reapply from the makeup we have in our set bags and it's usually not even the same color. Try something on and if it doesn't look good, tone it down. Mix colors. Be your own artist." Meg Thompson

Express Yourself

"There are no rules. Makeup is just about expressing your attitude and who you are. Apply makeup so that it represents you and makes you feel beautiful within and without. I love layering and mixing because the colors you can create by doing that are amazing." Galit Strugano

Sheer Perfection

"Look for sheer pigments. If you put it on your hand and can see through it, it's sheer. If it's too heavily pigmented, it will be old-fashioned and dated-looking. Sheerer pigments can look heavily pigmented in the container, but go on very sheer, and that's the way makeup is done today." Diane Gardner

Three Essentials

The three makeup items that every woman needs? It depends on who you ask. Terri Apanasewicz chooses "mascara, concealer, and lip color—lip color can double as cheek color," while for Napoleon Perdis, it's "mascara, lip gloss, and a good powder foundation to conceal, cover, and set," and for Peter Lamas, it's "lipstick, eyeliner, and concealer."

Lasting Beauty

"Makeup primers and sealants are on the rise. The Veil Foundation Primer from Bodyography is a fantastic primer. Also try SHE LAQ from Benefit to seal eyeliner and make it last all day." Terri Apanasewicz

Stay-Put Looks

"Work as closely as possible to your natural colors so when the makeup moves a bit, the look stays. Define lips with lipliner after applying your lipstick. Always use a shadow base to absorb oils on the eyes and help color stay true, and don't use a mascara that flakes." Napoleon Perdis

TIME-SAVERS

The Buzz from the Beauty Editor
Most of the time, multipurpose products don't work for me, but there's one notable exception: tinted moisturizer. My evening routine can be as extensive as I choose to make it, but I am not a morning person, so for a typical day of working at home on my computer or running errands, I look for ways to speed through my routine. I pick a tinted moisturizer with an SPF of at least 15 and some light, natural pigment. I can smooth it on when I'm still half-asleep and look reasonably polished with minimal effort.

Insider Information from the Beauty Bunch

Lifestyle Adjustments
"When my sister had kids, I started to take that into account in a lot of the things that I did. All of a sudden, a seventeen-step makeup routine and a twenty-step skin-care routine were no longer appropriate. They're wonderful if you have the time, but most people just want to be done with it. So it's important to take your lifestyle into account, even on a day-to-day basis. If you are going somewhere windy and you have long hair, then maybe MAC Lipglass isn't appropriate that day. There are no hard and fast rules. You don't have to spend hours a day to look beautiful." Stephen Sollitto

Multitasking
"Use single products for multiple purposes. Mix exfoliating cream with facial cleanser in your hand instead of using the two separately. As long as both foundation and moisturizer are water-based, they can be mixed together as well, or try a tinted moisturizer. Choose makeup with SPF and skip sunscreen." Giella

Quick Fix
Only got five minutes?

"Use concealer to spot cover and to brighten up eyes. Try a bit of lip color and blush to add that healthy color and brightness, and then use powder to set. Less can be more!" Terri Apanasewicz

"A bronzer, mascara, and lip gloss." Napoleon Perdis

Focus on a Feature
"A woman can look polished with only five minutes to apply her makeup by choosing to emphasize either her eyes or lips, and spending thirty seconds on one, and four and a half minutes on the other. If she's playing up her best feature, she'll look special." Peter Lamas

CONTOUR CLASS

The Buzz from the Beauty Editor
One of my best friends in high school had a body-image problem, and most of it centered around her face. Though she had long since lost her baby fat, her wide, square-shaped face remained, making her look, in her own words, "fat." She continued to diet, certain that someday her face would "catch up" to her body. What she didn't realize was that no amount of dieting would change her basic

bone structure. Only one thing could create the illusion of a smaller face: makeup. I pulled out a beauty book and some brown blush, and went to work contouring her face. My amateur efforts paid off, and when I twirled her around to face the mirror, her formerly boxy visage had taken on a newer, more streamlined shape. And she kicked the dieting habit. Not all self-image problems have such simple solutions, but this early experience opened my eyes to the transformative powers of makeup. Today, I use contouring only for special occasions, or when I am going to be photographed. I simply pick a brownish powder blush, a shade darker than my own color, apply sparingly, and blend like crazy.

Insider Information from the Beauty Bunch

Almost Perfect

"Create the illusion of perfection with contour and highlight. Contouring the face is the makeup artist's secret weapon for photography and evening light. The results can be transforming. When contouring, choose makeup a shade darker than your foundation. Be careful not to go too dark or it will look like dirt on your face. Highlighting will make any feature stand out and get noticed. When highlighting is used in conjunction with contour, the results are amazing." Debra Macki

Contour Correctly

"Most women want contoured cheekbones and the only way to do that is to trace your cheekbone up to the hairline using a darker shade. I usually use a tawny shade that doesn't have a lot of pink or red in it, like NARS Zen. It's almost like a bronzer. I follow the cheekbone with that and then, on just the apples of the cheeks, I use a fan-shaped brush to lightly apply a bright pink or red or apricot. I like MAC blush in Frankly Scarlet. It's a good contrast. I like the bronzer to contour and a light coat of the brighter color to brighten." Meg Thompson

Nose Jobs

"A wide nose can appear smaller by shading the sides and lightening the bridge. Apply contour shadow to the underside of the tip to shorten a long nose. Apply contour shadow in straight lines along the sides of the nose and a straight line of highlighter down the center to straighten a crooked nose." Debra Macki

Shape and Shade

"Skillful shading and highlighting helps enhance your best features and hide your less-desirable features. Understanding basic art techniques is essential. Light brings forward. Dark recedes. It is simple, but not always easy. Highlight cheekbones to make them more prominent. Use darker shades to contour or shadow underneath the cheekbones. This also makes them more prominent." Diane Ranger

Face It

"Oval face shapes need no corrective contour, but the natural bone structure can be enhanced more with a contour powder. Apply contour below cheekbone and under the jawline to give the illusion of a slimmer oval to a round face. For a square face, contour the widest part of the jaw and below the cheekbone, and contour the harsh square edges of the forehead to make it look more oval. If your face is heart-shaped, do not highlight cheekbones or use a bright cheek color. Shade the temples to narrow the top part of the face, and shade the tip of the chin. Highlight the mid-to-outer jawline. Diamond-shaped faces should also shun bright blush shades, and highlight the chin and forehead instead. Triangle-shaped faces can highlight each side of the forehead to create the illusion of width, pencil the eyebrows out slightly beyond the outer corners of the eyes, and minimize the jawline with contour." Debra Macki

Flaw Fixing

"High foreheads can be minimized by contouring along the hairline. Domed foreheads can be flattened by blending contour in the center section of the forehead to make it appear less round. To bring out a receding chin, highlight the tip." Debra Macki

GETTING YOUR GLOW ON

The Buzz from the Beauty Editor

A gorgeous glow is one of the God-given gifts of youth. Fortunately, it's easy to fake. The trick is in the application. Artfully applied, bronzers and highlighters leave you with a glow that seems to come from within. Misused, you look muddy (bronzer) or greasy (highlighter). The key with either is to apply very lightly, and only in the places where the light (or sun) would naturally hit your skin: along the temples, the bridge of the nose, the browbone, the tip of the chin, and the cheekbones. A dewy finish looks the most youthful, so steer clear of powder formulas and use creamy blushes and shadows.

Insider Information from the Beauty Bunch

Get a Glow

"Start with a hydrating moisturizer all over the face. These can be tinted for a very dewy look or followed with a foundation. Use powder lightly on T zone only. Blend highlighter on cheekbones and browbone for a luminous glow. For a very glowing look, spritz entire face with GIELLA Refining Vitamin C Tonic, which will also help set your makeup. You can also use a highlighting eye shadow to highlight cheekbones or browbones. A soft gold, white, or pink works very well." Giella

Multitask

"Always add a small dot of moisturizer to your foundation. It gives a beautiful glow and a wonderful slip to your product, and it keeps your skin dewy all day long." Dee DeLuca-Mattos

Buying Bronzer

"Test the bronzer around the feature focus of the face—nose, apples of cheeks, and forehead—and if it works well there, it will work well everywhere." Napoleon Perdis

Bronzer Setbacks

"Most bronzers absorb light and look just like clay on your face. Matte makes people look dull. It has to have reflective qualities; look for an ingredient like mica. Most people take bronzer and put it on their cheeks, the way you do a blush. That's not where it's supposed to go. It is supposed to be used on the forehead, nose, tops of cheeks, and a dab on the chin. Aside from the proper application, there is only one percent of the [female] population that looks good in bronzer: people with tanned bodies and pale faces, because you're matching your face to your body. I do think that bronzer is perfect for men." Diane Gardner

Star Quality

Glowing, starworthy skin can be achieved with "cream blush, powder through the T zone only, and lip gloss." Terri Apanasewicz

Glow On

"It's easy for makeup artists to give celebrities like Jennifer Lopez a natural-looking glow, because [they] take very good care of their skin. In other words, they already have a glow goin' on. Others who are not so lucky can benefit from a few subtle tricks, however. Always try to keep the foundation as close to the natural skintone as possible. If you go too dark, you look overdone. Too light, and you appear washed out. If you stick to your natural color, however, and use the base more to enhance than to cover, you'll look magical." Peter Lamas

Bronzed and Beautiful

"Instead of powder, use bronzer with a very light touch over makeup to set it. The glow is incredibly natural." Wende Zomnir

Bronze Bonanza

"Bronzers shouldn't have any orange in them. Cosmetic companies have a tendency to make orangey bronzers. Beware of coppers, which can look a little orange. Look for bronzers with some pink or peach in them. You want to look bronzed, but also like you've been out in the sun. A combination of gold, pink, and bronze [all together] in a bronzer will help you look as if you've been in the sun. The intensity of the bronzer has a lot to do with the person's skin color to begin with; if you are really fair, you can look bronzed with a very light color. I like bronzers in powder or cream or liquid; it

depends on what the client likes and the application. If you don't need to wear foundation, a liquid or cream bronzer is great. With foundation, it's better to use a powder. And I do like a little shimmer because it's light reflective, but you don't need much. A little bit goes a long way." Bobbe Joy

Hurry Up and Glow

"Use a primer, such as Napoleon Perdis Auto Pilot, to infuse and reactivate skin care. Work prominent features with a loose, iridescent dust and use powder only in the areas [you] don't want reflection." Napoleon Perdis

The Highlights of Highlighter

"I love highlighting creams. The ones with pigment look the most natural. NARS Multiples are my favorites. I use Copacabana every day down the bridge of my nose and under the browbone. You can use them as your blush instead of adding a crystal-white highlighter at the end, on top of your blush, which can look too placed. I like to highlight with MAC loose highlighting powder, the only kind I use, when I'm done with my makeup. I use the Shu Uemura #14H brush, which is like a slanted blush brush but half the size, and dip it into the top of the loose highlighting powder and tap off the excess. Then I make a "C" shape, sort of like a boomerang, from above the eyebrow at the end of the arch, then trace it over the bone and around, stopping just over the apple of the cheek. You should end in a straight line down from where you started above the brow. If it's fine enough, it won't look like glitter or shimmer; it will look dewy." Meg Thompson

Hints on Highlighters

"I like a silicone-based highlighter that is very light-reflective and that doesn't get in the cracks and crevices. Use just a drop on your fingertip and apply it to the upper part of the cheekbone and take it all the way under your eye. Powders are also easy to use: sweep some on the upper portion of your cheekbone and bring it around the eye a little bit. Be careful that they don't have too much frost in them, or they can accentuate your wrinkles. When picking a highlighter color, I try not to use white because that can get a little scary. It can be a light soft gold or beige gold or soft beigey pink. Those are probably the best colors, the ones that look good on most people. You can also use a really light bronzer as a highlighter; just make sure it doesn't get too dark." Bobbe Joy

Bronzed Definition

"I always apply a little bronzer or contour to define the face. I start from underneath the cheekbone next to the ear and brush toward the apple of the cheeks. Next, I swipe the brush to the temples and release the remaining bronzer to the rest of the face. This technique allows for a more natural bronze look to the face." Lilly Rivera

Easy Glow

"Use a stick foundation as a highlighter on whatever features you want to bring out, such as browbone, bridge of nose, top of lip, cheekbones, and around lipliner." Napoleon Perdis

THE FOUNDATION FILES

The Buzz from the Beauty Editor

I'm a little obsessed with finding the right foundation, and I think many women share the same fixation. I have high hopes for a makeup base: it needs to provide coverage while still letting my natural skintone and texture show through; it needs to last all day without settling into creases and fine lines; and, of course, it needs to be a perfect match for my skin color.

Insider Information from the Beauty Bunch

Foundation Tips

"When you're shopping for foundation, try to match your skintone in natural sunlight. Apply a strip of foundation to your skin without blending; if it changes color, it's the wrong shade. Look for a color that disappears into your skin. How you apply foundation depends on your personal preference. If you prefer using sponges, a polyurethane sponge is best, as opposed to latex, since it is softer and can be reused after washing with a gentle soap. Pour a small amount of foundation onto the back of your hand and dip your sponge into the foundation. Next, dab the sponge on your forehead, cheeks, chin, and nose, blending outward. (Wash sponges thoroughly with an antibacterial cleanser after each use, rinse well, and then pop in microwave to dry. Germs love moisture.)

"The same applies when using your fingertips— use your ring finger and middle finger to blend foundation from your nose to your cheek and down the jawline. Just remember to wash your hands first with an antibacterial soap. If you choose a brush for blending foundation, synthetic brushes with a two-inch head work best. Apply five dots of foundation on each area of your face and blend outward. Remember to wash brushes with gentle soap after each use. If your foundation cakes up, try another brand. However, you can also try to apply it very lightly. Use foundation where needed, and [keep it] very sheer on the rest of your face." Giella

Tool Time
"A foundation brush is better for applying makeup because it puts the smallest amount of makeup exactly where you want it." Bobbe Joy

Spendworthy
"Splurge on foundation." Napoleon Perdis

Flawed Foundation
"The most common mistake women make with their makeup is using the wrong shade of foundation. It's so unattractive when the skin color appears to change at the neck." Peter Lamas

Face Base
"For a more flawless and smoother makeup application, I apply a thin coat of Hyaluronic Acid serum as a primer before makeup. It holds over one thousand times its weight in water, plumps the skin, smoothes out fine lines and wrinkles, and improves the texture of the skin. It is considered a super moisturizer, and it can be used as an anti-aging night treatment." Lilly Rivera

Olive Branches
"Olive-skinned people often have a tough time getting the right shade of foundation, because a lot of olive or sallow-skinned women get categorized as yellow-orange, which is incorrect. But that's because many makeup lines have two main categories: yellow-orange or blue-red. The common problem with the foundation colors available is that they don't address the majority of skintones, which are yellow-based with a blue undertone (olive). There are many yellow-based foundations on the market, but not many that are yellow-blue. Ninety percent of my customers fall into this yellow-blue category." Giella

Easy Application
"Apply liquid foundation with your hands, the way you would apply a moisturizer, and rub it into skin for a flawless finish." Mala Elhassan

Finding Foundation
"It's really important to have good lighting. One of the problems at a department store is that you feel pressure to decide quickly, and the lighting is usually not good. First, pick a shade that is lighter or darker than your skintone so that you can see the foundation on your hand, the contrast on your skin. Play with the texture on your hand, and watch how it settles into your pores. Walk around with it. Smell it. A lot of lines smell like sunscreen, which is not a problem because its important for me to have sunscreen in my foundation, but a lot of them smell too musty or too much like makeup. After you decide that you like the way it feels and smells, have the salesperson put [the closest shade] on you and wear it around that day when you are shopping. Go outside with it on. You don't necessarily want to buy it right away. Things look different when they've been on your skin for a while. Your foundation will also look different as your skin changes, which it will, according to your diet or how hydrated you are." Meg Thompson

Foundation Foibles
"I just had a woman come in here saying how hard it is to pick the right foundation in a department store. You go into the store and you don't know about the products, and you are relying on someone else to tell you about them, and you wind up buying the wrong thing. You can't put it on your hand to test it; you have to put it on the spot between the chin and the

neck. I see women take it and put it on their hand, but the hand has nothing to do with the face. And you have to walk outside with it on. Don't rely on the lighting in [the] makeup department. Also, make sure that you pick the right type of foundation for your skin type. As you get older, your foundation needs to be more light-reflective. If you use a matte foundation on older skin, it highlights the cracks and crevices. You don't want to use all oil-free products if your skin is dehydrated, because it will look flat. The makeup doesn't necessarily need to have oil in it, but it needs to have some type of hydration. And then there are the people with beautiful skin, who don't need foundation at all, maybe just a tinted moisturizer and a stick foundation on spots that need more coverage." Bobbe Joy

Foundation Feats

"When I am applying foundation on other people I use a brush, but when I'm doing my own makeup I warm up the foundation on the top of my hand first. I never put it directly from the tube to the face. If you apply a swatch of the foundation on the back of your hand, and apply the pigment from there, you'll find that you use less product, which is a good thing. When you're done, you usually have some left on your hand." Meg Thompson

Foundation Foul-Up

"One mistake women make is using foundation that is too dark, so that it looks like a head sitting on someone else's body. Sometimes celebrities do this because the flash from the camera actually bleaches out the skintone. Someone I know saw Jessica Simpson out at a party, and her makeup was so orange and so dark, but it looked fabulous in pictures. She did that intentionally because she's flashed so much." Bobbe Joy

First Base

"Always test the foundation on the cheek, not near the jawline. Always use a foundation shade on the warmer side." Napoleon Perdis

Foolproof Foundation

"To apply foundation, I use a wet sponge saturated with warm water. I mix a little moisturizer into the foundation, and I apply that mixture with the wet sponge. Foundation tends to be too heavy for me unless the person has really bad acne; otherwise, I do a light application on everybody. I don't think you need as much coverage as the cosmetic companies want you to have. I tap the sponge all over the skin, pressing it into the skin. This method is sort of like sponging a wall; if you sponged enough you would cover the wall but the look would be softer. With this method, there are no hard lines. With some foundations, if you apply them in a conventional way, you just see streak lines, but with this method I can use practically any foundation on anybody." Stephen Sollitto

CONCEALER CUES

The Buzz from the Beauty Editor

I've got a lot to hide. That's why I consider concealer an absolute essential. Many times, I'll slip it on over moisturizer, add a light dusting of powder, and head out the door, foundation-free. Concealer can look cakey and unnatural if used incorrectly. Here's a great tip I picked up from a friend. The moment you step out of the shower, while skin is still moist, apply concealer just where you need it, over your skin-care products. By the time you're ready to tackle your makeup, your concealer will have sunk in, and you'll be left with nothing but natural coverage.

Insider Information from the Beauty Bunch

Taking Cover

"Don't cover up an entire undereye circle. Apply a sort of inverted triangle of concealer in the inner corner of the eye. Never swim it around so there's a sea of light concealer under the eye. I like to apply foundation first all over the face, even under the eye, and then go back and touch up. I used to do it the other way and it seemed I was wiping off all the coverup. Now I just touch up where I need to touch up. You'll be amazed at what your foundation covers up." Stephen Sollitto

Conceal and Seal

"To keep your lips and eyes intact, a great concealer—I love Sebastian Trucco—on lips, eyes, even a little on cheeks, keeps everything in place all day." Dee DeLuca-Mattos

Lighten Up

"A lot of people want to lighten the dark circles under their eyes, which only highlights them. Dark shades push back while light shades enhance. You want to push back your dark circles, not accentuate them, so you should choose a concealer color that is almost the same color as your skin, with the right undertone. Mix eye cream with your concealer, and you will get more of a hydrated look." Giella

Ingenious Idea

"I wear a shade darker in my concealer than my foundation, which sounds a little weird, but be wary of a concealer that is too light. It only makes the circles more obvious. I always apply a little pressed or loose powder over the concealer." Meg Thompson

Which Comes First?

"It shouldn't matter whether you use a concealer first or foundation first, because your concealer shouldn't be so light that you have to blend it into your foundation. It should be able to stand on its own." Giella

THE POWDER ROOM

The Buzz from the Beauty Editor

Powder is so essential, and yet it's also tricky. Artfully applied, it sets makeup and blots shine. When misused, it can make foundation look splotchy and wrinkles more pronounced. I always use a light touch, and wait a few minutes after applying foundation to add powder. Otherwise, it will stick to moist patches of skin, making it look blotchy and muddy, and making your application seem heavy-handed. Once foundation dries, powder goes on much more smoothly and looks more natural.

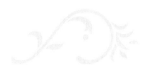

Inside Information from the Beauty Bunch

Perfecting Powder

"I don't usually put a lot of powder on, except in the T zone. I prefer to use a loose translucent powder. It shouldn't be so pigmented that it settles in and makes your foundation look like a different color. Whenever I apply powder, whether with a brush or a sponge, I brush it off on the top of my hand before applying it. Otherwise, it can look uneven. Sometimes, uneven application comes from the way the powder is attaching to the brush or sponge. If it's already cakey on the sponge, it will be cakey on your face. This is true for any powder application, whether it's eye shadow, blush, or face powder. I use my brush and tap it onto the skin. I stipple it." Meg Thompson

Obliterate the Oilies

"Very oily skin should be dusted with a finishing powder before applying any other product. Finish your makeup, and then add another dusting of finishing powder. Set with a spritzer." Diane Ranger

Hold the Powder

"An older woman should use as little powder as possible. She should only put it in the areas where she is going to use another form of powder makeup. If she's wearing powder blush or eye shadow, she should just put powder on her eyelids and her cheeks. Never apply powder with a sponge; if you do, you are really applying a lot of powder and pressing it onto the skin so that it looks cakey. Use a big fluffy brush and just lay on the lightest amount. Use a synthetic brush, because that's the kind of brush that will lay the makeup onto the skin rather than absorbing it or messing up your foundation. A sponge is absorbent, and it lays down the color with-

out any of the moisture that you need to spread the product around properly. A sponge is great for blending. We use it on TV to blot out the oil on the cracks on the sides of the nose. I never use powder puffs in real life—only on a film set, when you need to apply a lot of product. In the real world, you would look extremely made up. You don't want to look extremely made up. You just want to look good." Bobbe Joy

Powder Pick

"Use a powder that matches your foundation." Napoleon Perdis

Fabulous Finish

"For a soft focus finish, brush on a finishing powder. Always spritz the mineral makeup with a Colorescience Achromatherapy Gem Spritzer to 'set' the makeup. This gives a soft dewy look and ensures longer wear." Diane Ranger

Once Over Lightly

"To set foundation, I use T. LeClerc Loose Powder in Banane on most skintones. Using the Shu Uemura No. 16 brush, which is a smaller brush, I dust the powder on very lightly, tapping not wiping. On darker skin, I use MAC Studio Fix C5 or C6 with an even lighter touch, because Studio Fix has some coverage. I hardly ever put powder under the eyes, because that's where the lines are and the skin is very delicate, so it gets cakey very quickly. After I'm done with the powder on the rest of the face, I will sometimes take what's left on the brush, which is usually nothing, and tap it under the eyes. You always have to go very lightly under the eyes because the more makeup you have, the more you will accentuate the lines. That's why I like to use moisturizer and a very light application." Stephen Sollitto

THE BEAUTY OF BLUSH

The Buzz from the Beauty Editor
When I was a teenager, my mother never let me out of the house without blush and earrings. After temporarily falling out of favor with me in the early nineties, I'm hooked on blush again. Nothing brightens, freshens, or gives a more youthful glow than the right blush.

Insider Information from the Beauty Bunch

Blushing Basics

"Don't apply blush too close to your eyes. Leave a two-finger-width space between your eye and the start of your blush. Start in the middle of your pupil and blend to the middle of your ear, always leaving that two-finger space. Blush is too far up if it sits on top of your cheekbone. It should sit on and below the bone. Try softening the edges and setting blush with a light dusting of powder. Powder typically gives a drier, matte look, and creams and tints give a more hydrated look. Cheek tints have become very popular as they are lightweight and easy to apply. They give a wash of color with a very natural glow. For oily skin types, or those with acne, stick with powder blush, but dry dehydrated skin types can try the creams or tints. Cheekbones can be more pronounced with the proper color and placement of blush." Giella

How to Blush

"A good rounded blush brush—it can even be used with cream blush—is essential for perfect application. Concentrate on the apples of the cheeks and blend out. Think about where we really blush in a natural situation and mimic it." Terri Apanasewicz

Blush Beautifully

"The ideal method for applying blush is to first look in the mirror, and smile. This will help you see which area of your face you are trying to highlight. If you are using powder blush, start at the apple of your cheek, and gently brush up your cheekbone toward your hairline. If you are using cream blush, dot it beginning at the apple, and gently blend up the cheekbone toward the hairline." Peter Lamas

Pointers for Picking Blush

"Blush should complement your lips. Depending on the lip color, blush should be in the same shade: brown/bronze, peach/orange, coral/red, pink/fuchsia or plum/berry. However, there are some shades of blush with equal parts of brown, orange, red, pink, and plum that work well with most lip colors. Colors that are brighter, such as a rose or peach, are great accents to highlight cheekbones. Darker (browner) colors will make cheekbones recede and should not be used. Also, try some soft shimmer over your blush, like GIELLA Lust Dust, for an added lift to the cheekbone. Colors that contain a little bit of everything—red, pink, brown, and orange—will go with a variety of skin colors. If you have light hair, from light brown to blonde to strawberry blonde, and any eye color, go for a brown shade with a medium value—not too dark or too light. Women with dark hair and eyes can't use blush that is too muted or muddy; they need deeper shades." Giella

Blush Blunder

"The second-biggest mistake, after using a bronzer on your cheeks instead of blush, is choosing a blush color that's not bright enough. A lot of people go for the old-fashioned violet blushes, or pinks with a violet base, out of habit. They are afraid, so they don't pick the bright apricot that would look great on them." Diane Gardner

Blushing Double

"I like to use a bronzer and a blush at the same time. I use a bronze color first, all over, because it looks more real, and then apply pink blush on top of it, right on the apples of the cheeks. To choose a blush shade, I first determine what color tones I am going to use all over the face, because the blush has to go with the rest of the makeup. I pick a colorway based on the person's skintone, so the whole look blends beautifully. For example, for a redhead with some yellow in her skin, I am probably not going to use taupes on her; I am going to use warmer colors, not cool ones. I might use a golden peach on lids, a lighter version of that shade under the browbone, some nutmeg in the crease, and a peachy-gold blush. So it all ends up blending together really softly and giving you that all-over tone. Sometimes you need a lot more color. If the client needs color, I would add some bronze to it, if her skin were darker, but keep it in the same tone. I wouldn't do a red or pink blush with the peach makeup, for example. It starts to look like a circus on your face." Bobbe Joy

Faking It

"Blush should be applied like the sun has kissed you. Start at the apple of the cheek and sweep up towards the edge of the eye. Use a firm blush brush or feather brush." Napoleon Perdis

Lush and Rosy

"When using a cream, it's best to use a sheer berry-pink or red color to look glowing but not severe. Avoid orange, brick, and fuchsia, or colors that are too matte and too deep. If you are using a powder blush, use one with a slight sheen in it. For example, a subtle gold or white shimmer makes the cheek look more luminous. For application, focus more on the apples of the cheeks rather then sharp diagonals that are best for contouring. Lush rosy cheeks look best in a circular motion, blending upward to the inner ear. Blend with your ring finger, which has the least amount of pressure on your face, to avoid applying color too heavily." Giella

Blushing Beauty

"I do agree with some people who say that the placement of blush should be the hollows of the cheeks, but I like to tap it on and not drag it back and forth. When you drag on your blusher, there's more of a definitive line, but if you stipple it back and forth, it's a more muted, softer edge. I like to add a darker color to the hollows of the cheeks and a lighter version of that color to the apple to give it a little dimension so there's not just one color on the cheek. But this is for people who love to do it—some women do not want to spend that kind of time. There is some unwritten rule that blush is not supposed to be up close to the eye, but with the right coloring, I do bring it up there because if you're flushed, sometimes you will have color there, especially if I am using a lighter color. I don't necessarily bring the color in the hollow of the cheek all the way back; I do leave some space between the hairline and the hollow." Stephen Sollitto

Cheeky Blusher

"To enhance the cheekbones, apply a dark or subtle shade of taupe blush, depending on your skintone, underneath the cheekbone. Be conservative; too much may make you look hollow and give you an aged look. Add a highlighter on the top of the cheek to bring out the bone, then swipe the remaining highlighter on the center of the face to bring it forward." Lilly Rivera

Blush Selection

"The shade of blush you choose depends on your skintone. Women with olive skin can wear a lot of different things. For a woman with very fair skin, a shade of red that is too dark may not be appropriate, but a paler pink might work. But if your hair is blonde, you might need more red because you might need some color. I am a firm believer that the trick is in your application. Even if you're using the wrong color, if you're using a sheer-enough application, you can put anything on your face. Stick your finger in it at the store before you dismiss it, because I've often initially dismissed colors that turned out to be great." Stephen Sollitto

THE PRODUCT FILES

Foundations

The Buzz from the Beauty Editor

I prefer to apply foundation with my fingers, because the warmth of your body heat liquifies the product, making application easier and the look more natural. Another great option is to use a foundation brush. (Paula Dorf gave me this tip, and hers is exceptional.) It seems to blend foundation into skin more lightly and evenly, creating flawless coverage. For extra coverage, dab your foundation on rather than rubbing it in. Some of my favorite foundations include Giorgio Armani Luminous Silk Foundation, $52.50, and Shu Uemura Nobara Cream Foundation, $24.

What the Pros Choose

The pros pick foundation formulas ranging from popular favorites to little-known names. Mala Elhassan and Lilly Rivera both choose MAC, with Rivera specifying Studio Fix and Elhassan citing Face and Body, while June Jacobs and Julie Hewett both pick Laura Mercier. "I love that it's hydrating and oil-free," Hewett raves. "The colors are perfect!" Wende Zomnir picks Urban Decay Surreal Skin Liquid Makeup, Shauna Raisch chooses Aveda Inner Light Dual Foundation SPF 12, and Hara Glick loves Sue Devitt Seaweed Foundation. Danielle Browning has two favorites: Trish McEvoy Even Skin and Lola Oil-Free Creme Foundation. Meg Thompson also has two picks. About her current favorite, Stephane Marais Crème Foundation, Thompson says that "it looks dark when you put it on and then settles into the skin and ends up being the right color. My friends and I are all going one shade darker than we thought we would." Thompson also loves Bobbi Brown, because the "the colors are great and not at all ashy." Cult favorites include Il Makiage Professional Studio Creme Makeup (in IM-M10, picked by Galit Strugano), Trucco Duo Powder Foundation (Dee DeLuca-Mattos), Pharmaskincare (Meredith Green), Cinema Secrets Ultimate Foundation (Debra Luftman), Lavera Makeup Fluid (Linda Deslauriers), and Giorgio Armani Luminous Silk Foundation (a second pick from Lilly Rivera).

Concealers

The Buzz from the Beauty Editor

I look for a product that matches my skintone, blends in effortlessly, and stays inconspicuous. When I'm wearing foundation, I apply concealer after the foundation. Often, my base covers almost everything, and I need only a minimal amount of concealer. I love Laura Mercier Secret Camouflage, $28, and MAC Select Concealer, $13.

What the Pros Choose

Hara Glick and Lilly Rivera love Laura Mercier Secret Concealer, while June Jacobs and Julie Hewett both choose Yves Saint Laurent as the best way to take cover. Hewett also singles out Joe Blasco; Wende Zomnir picks Urban Decay Urban Camouflage Concealer; Shauna Raisch likes Aveda Inner Light Concealer in Balsa; and Galit Strugano chooses Cinema Secrets. Debra Macki picks her own Camouflage Cover Crème; Mala Elhassan picks Vincent Longo Cream Concealer; and Dee DeLuca-Mattos loves Sebastian Trucco. Meg Thompson reaches for Bobbi Brown Creamy Concealer. "It gives a lot of coverage, lasts forever, and the pots screw together. You can blend them according to your skintone." In stick form, her pick is Stephane Marais.

Powders

The Buzz from the Beauty Editor

I always keep a pressed-powder compact in my bag. It can freshen makeup in a flash, and a beautiful powder compact is a classic, feminine accessory. But pressed powder can be overused. I always try blotting papers first, to soak up excess oil. Sometimes they're enough to do the trick. If I feel more coverage or shine prevention is called for, I pull out the pressed powder, which goes on much more smoothly over skin that's just been blotted. I apply sparingly, and avoid the eye area, where it can accentuate fine lines. My favorite loose powders are Becca Fine Loose

Finishing Powder, $38, and L'Oreal Visible Lift Line Minimizing Powder, $12. In pressed form, I love Hard Candy O-blot-erate, $16, and Lola Pressed Powder, $27.50.

What the Pros Choose

In the loose-powder category, two of our pros pick MAC (June Jacobs and Dee DeLuca-Mattos). Julie Hewett stands by the classic T. LeClerc in Banane; Meg Thompson chooses Armani; Debra Luftman picks Cinema Secrets; and Shauna Raisch likes Aveda Inner Light Loose Powder. For pressed powders, Galit Strugano chooses MAC in NC45; Julie Hewett loves T. LeClerc in Banane; June Jacobs prefers Laura Mercier; Shauna Raisch picks Aveda Inner Light Pressed Powder in Honey; Meg Thompson chooses LORAC; Dee DeLuca-Mattos picks Shu Uemura; and Mala Elhassan likes Make Up For Ever.

Bronzers/Highlighters

The Buzz from the Beauty Editor

For a starworthy glow, start with an eye cream, followed by concealer to brighten shadows around the eyes. Then apply foundation mixed with a little highlighting cream (like Benefit High Beam, $20, or LORAC Oil-Free Luminizer, $28) only on areas that need coverage, and follow with a cream or gel blush (Tarte Cheek Stain, $28, or NARS The Multiple, $36) in a rosy shade. Apply creamy shadow in a pearly shade (like Bloom Sheer Color Cream in Glow, $15) all over lid. If you must finish with a powder, use a brush and the lightest possible touch, and avoid fine lines. Try an ultrasheer translucent or highlighting powder, like Revlon SkinLights Face Illuminator Powder Brightener, $12.

What the Pros Choose

The pros are divided between bronzers and high-lighters. On the bronzer side, there is Wende Zomnir (Urban Decay Bronzing Powder in Baked), Napoleon Perdis (Napoleon Perdis Mosaic Bronzer), Julie Hewett (Christian Dior Terra Bella Sun Powder), Dee DeLuca-Mattos (Prescriptives Sunsheen Bronzing Gel), Danielle Browning (Tarte Pressed Blush in Ra), Fiona Locke (California Tan Suddenly Sun Bronzing Powder—Locke loves that the single shade works on everyone), and Shauna Raisch (Aveda Petal Essence Face Accents in Bronze Glow). Pros who pick one of each include Galit Strugano (Pretty Pretty Face & Body Bronzing Powder in D'orazia and Girlactik Beauty Chic Shine in Starlet Pink) and Lilly Rivera (BridalGal Mosaic Bronzing Powder and Mosaic Gleamer). For a cream bronzer, Meg Thompson loves NARS Multiple in Copacabana, and in a powder, she chooses Becca Pressed Bronzing Powder. Thompson also loves MAC Iridescent Powder/Loose in Silver Dusk. NARS was also Mala Elhassan's pick. Other pros who pick highlighters include Napoleon Perdis (Napoleon Perdis Loose Dust in Sand Beige), Hara Glick (Clinique Colour Rub Allover Lustre), and Meredith Green (Benefit High Beam and Revlon SkinLights Instant Skin Brightener, which she says "brightens even the dullest complexion, and makes skin look dewy and fresh").

Blush

The Buzz from the Beauty Editor

For a natural, everyday look, I smile and apply rosy blush just to the apples of my cheeks. It instantly perks up my complexion. Keep it away from the undereye area, though; it will just look messy. My favorites are Stila Blush Duo in Cruise to Cairo, $28, Tarte Cheek Stain in Tickled Peach, $28, and Physicians Formula Planet Blush, $11.

What the Pros Choose

In the blush category, the winning pick is Stila, chosen by Dee DeLuca-Mattos and Julie Hewett (Stila Cream Blush). Other favorites include MAC (June Jacobs), Benefit Benetint (Mala Elhassan), Aveda Petal Essence Cheek Color in Apricot Glow (Shauna Raisch), Hard Candy Sweet Cheeks in Sugar (Wende Zomnir), NARS Orgasm (Hara Glick), Lola One Night Stand (Galit Strugano), and Trish McEvoy Tangerine Glow (Danielle Browning). Meg Thompson has three picks: in cream form, she loves NARS Multiple in Cannes and Prescriptives Creamy Cheekcolor in any shade, because they're all "beautiful." In a powder, she likes NARS Powder Blush Cheek Color in Torrid.

Chapter Four

Beauty School:
Face-Saving Secrets Only the Pros Know

The truly beauty-obsessed, like myself, always want to be on top of the next big thing. That's why I am so fascinated by mineral and airbrushed makeup. They are entirely new categories. For years, foundation choices remained pretty much the same: pancake, cream, and liquid formulations were our only options. Now, new types of products mean new techniques. Even if you don't consider yourself a beauty addict, the information on these pages can help you win friends and influence people. Or, at the very least, simplify your makeup routine and clear up a few misconceptions. By the end, you too will be a beauty insider.

THE *Beauty Bunch* BREAKDOWN

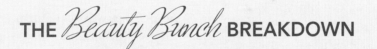

Napoleon Perdis: Australian celebrity makeup artist with an eponymous makeup line.

Kari Boatner: permanent-cosmetics pioneer who has developed innovative instruments and artistic procedures for the application of permanent makeup.

Terri Apanasewicz: celebrity makeup artist with L.A.'s Cloutier Agency whose clients have included Michael Michele, Jeri Ryan, Kristin Davis, Toni Braxton, and Reba McEntire.

Meg Thompson: Hollywood makeup artist and co-owner/founder of Madge Cosmetics.

Peter Lamas: founder and chairman of Lamas Beauty International, a rapidly growing, well-respected natural beauty product manufacturer.

Giella: Professional makeup artist and founder of GIELLA Custom Blend Cosmetics.

Debra Macki: a top Boston-based makeup artist and the founder of Debra Macki Cosmetics.

Diane Ranger: the founder of mineral makeup, and the founder and owner of Colorescience Cosmetics.

Lilly Rivera: celebrated makeup artist at the prestigious Dominique Salon in the Hotel Pierre, New York City.

Hollis Wright: makeup artist and skin-care expert with over twenty years of experience.

Bobbe Joy: celebrity makeup artist whose clients include Lucy Liu, Scarlett Johansson, Naomi Watts, Jennifer Tilly, and Janice Dickinson, she also has a signature line of products, Makeup! Bobbe Joy.

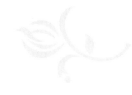

AGE-ERASING MAKEUP

The Buzz from the Beauty Editor

Time travel is possible with the right makeup. The key to youthful beauty? Moderation. Overdoing your makeup is instantly aging, but so is skipping makeup altogether. Steer clear of powders and opt for creamy formulations, particularly around the eye area. Also, cut your concealer with a little eye cream to keep it from settling into the fine lines around the eyes. Finally, don't forget to blush. A dab of rosy color on the apples of the cheeks is the single quickest way to a younger, fresher appearance.

Insider Information from the Beauty Bunch

Look Five Years Younger

In Your 20s: "Use a tinted moisturizer with a high-lighting powder, in gold or white, to even out skin-tone and cover blemishes. Give your eyes a punch with a sheer wash of color to brighten your eyes; for example, a blue-gold works great for brown, green, and blue eyes. Definitely opt for a shiny lip with lip gloss, and avoid dark lipliner. Use a liner that blends in with your lip color."

In Your 30s: "Try using a cheek tint rather than a powder blush. Cheek tints provide a sheer wash of color on the cheeks that gives a radiant, youthful glow. Don't forget to use an eye-shadow primer to cover the darkness, veins, capillaries, and shadows above your eyes, not just below. It should cover the skin from the eyelid up to the brow. When lip color starts settling in the fine lines, it is time for a lip primer that will help plump up fine lines and keep the color from settling in the 'cracks,' especially for smokers."

In Your 40s: "Light-reflecting powders, shimmers, and lotions are the answer to making skin glow. They bring light to the skin without looking too glittery or frosty. Brow tints are the perfect way to cover gray eyebrows. As we age, our brows get lighter and turn gray. The brow tints are applied daily to coat the hairs without looking too heavy or 'done.' Choose a shade that complements your hair color or a shade lighter. Avoid using a lip color that is too dark—brighter colors can really be more uplifting. If you are used to using browns, try lightening them with a pink, red, or orange color in a lip pencil or lipstick." Giella

De-Age Your Makeup

"The two biggest mistakes mature women make are wearing too much makeup and not wearing any makeup. Older women have trouble wearing warm colors because they only accentuate the sallow cast of a mature complexion. A general rule is to draw attention away from a troubled area by playing it down and emphasizing a positive feature.

"The foundation that worked at twenty-five is not going to do the trick at forty. Outdated colors and styles will make you look older than you are. Too much foundation accentuates wrinkles; use a thinner foundation on older skin. If foundation does not sit smoothly on the face, use a sponge for even coverage and make sure to exfoliate for better makeup application. Do not attempt to use foundation to hide expression lines. Makeup cannot hide them and will accentuate the problem instead of covering it. Draw attention to a positive feature instead.

"Use a very light touch with concealer, because it is noticeable in lines. Use a light foundation instead, if possible, and apply moisturizer first to act as filler. Too much powder, incorrectly applied, will bring out wrinkles and make you look older. If your powder is magnifying your wrinkles and making your face look cakey, apply it with a sponge so you have more control of where it's going, and avoid wrinkled areas. But powder is essential, because shine accentuates wrinkles too. Apply it correctly. If your face is thinning, apply blush to the apples of cheeks to give the illusion of a fuller face, and do not contour. Lips lose contour with age, and lipliner can make a big difference." Debra Macki

Age-Defying Application

"Blush and concealer in just the right places [can make you look younger]—over-application will actually age you. Nothing is better than blush for adding a healthy glow. For skin care, moisturizer [is essential] to keep skin youthful." Terri Apanasewicz

Conceal Your Age

"A good concealer under the eyes can work wonders for taking years off your appearance." Peter Lamas

Youth-Oriented

"Lining the inner corner of the eye gives an instant eye lift. Do not apply foundation to forehead; just apply a light dusting of powder. Always wear polish on fingers and toes to deflect your age. Smooth on a reflective body moisturizer." Napoleon Perdis

SPECIAL AGENTS:
MINERAL, AIRBRUSHED, AND PERMANENT MAKEUP

The Buzz from the Beauty Editor

When I started wearing foundation, there were only a few formulas available: thick liquids, creams, or pancake makeup. Now, the options are virtually limitless, and each offers something unique. If you're looking for complete, waterproof coverage that feels and looks virtually invisible, try the new airbrush foundations. With a little practice, these formulas offer amazing, lasting coverage. Looking for something a little easier to apply? Try mineral makeup. Unlike standard foundations, mineral makeup foundations are powders that feel creamy when applied. They brush on easily to create even, weightless, foolproof coverage. Plus, they're water-resistant and contain an SPF of 15 or higher. Finally, for the most lasting fix of all, try micropigmentation, or permanent makeup. If you are so fair that you appear washed out until you apply your eyeliner and brow pencil, or if you simply want to save time and effort, then permanent makeup may be your best bet.

Insider Information from the Beauty Bunch

Matching Your Minerals
"You choose a mineral makeup in exactly the way they tell you not to with traditional makeup. You test it on the inside of your arm. Mineral makeup adapts to your skintone so you can't make a really serious mistake. There's good and then there's better. If it disappears, it's the perfect color. If you have to ask if it's too dark or light, too warm or cool, then it's not the right shade." Diane Ranger

Addicted to Airbrushing
"Airbrushed makeup, like the kind made by Kett Cosmetics, allows for a beautiful, flawless, smudge-resistant look in person as well as in digital or high-definition photography, without the heavy feel or look. Airbrushed blush looks much more natural, as if it comes from within. Layer with a light dusting of powder to set. The results are gorgeous and flawless-looking for eight hours with very minimal touch-ups." Lilly Rivera

Signed, Sealed, Delivered
"If you insist on a technician who is board certified by the American Academy of Micropigmentation, this ensures that he or she is a professional who has received extensive training and is committed to the field, and not someone who received a certificate for an hour-long course. Don't use money as a criterion when choosing a permanent-cosmetics professional. You are better off not doing it at all. Quality varies widely, which is why it's important that you choose a qualified specialist. Micropigmentation (permanent makeup) is virtually unregulated in this country. Anyone can say that they are a certified technician, but that means nothing unless they are board certified by the A.A.M. For example, there are only sixty board-certified technicians in the state of Florida, but there are hundreds of technicians practicing without board certification." Kari Boatner

Mastering Mineral Makeup
"In some ways, mineral makeup is the opposite of conventional makeup. With conventional makeup, you usually put on a pigmented cream or liquid foundation and then a sheer powder to set it. But with mineral makeup, the cream (like Colorescience F.A.C.E. Crème de la Creme) is a sheer primer, for lifting and shaping and evening the skintone. I developed the primers in my forties, when, for the first time, my mineral makeup was not lasting through the day. It's the powder that has the pigment. You shouldn't apply too much of the powder at once. Use light layers, but as many layers as you want, to avoid a heavy, cakey look. That heavy look is the biggest complaint, but that's because people apply too much.

"Too much makeup gives you the cadaver look, but these minerals are meant to make your skin look young and alive and bright, like they're backlit, and not drab. If you see makeup, it's too much, and if it feels like something's on then there's something wrong. It should feel like you have nothing on. It's ideal for anyone who hates the feel of makeup. When these products were first launched, we had a little trouble convincing women in Texas and Georgia, because they were so used to the feel of makeup, but once they got used to it they never went back." Diane Ranger

COLOR THEORY

The Buzz from the Beauty Editor

I've always found color selection to be the most challenging aspect of makeup application, until I developed my very own, highly unscientific system for choosing and using colors. I simply wear what I love. If my current obsession is red lipstick, I wear red lipstick. Any woman can wear red, or any color, for that matter; the key is in the shade she chooses. I look to my wardrobe and my home for inspiration, because I believe that most of us instinctively choose the colors that suit us best. Finally, I try the color on. Does it look amazing, or just all right? Do my teeth look whiter, my eyes brighter? If a color doesn't wow me, I pass. If it does, I am unfailingly loyal.

Insider Information from the Beauty Bunch

The Age Factor
"We all see color differently, and our perception of color changes as we age. As we get older, we see more yellow. That's why older people are more attracted to clearer, brighter colors." Hollis Wright

Buy What You Love
To choose makeup colors that suit you, try "color therapy—choosing colors you are drawn to." Or splurge on a "one-on-one consultation with a make-up artist." Napoleon Perdis

Swatch Selection
"Shopping for makeup shades is like shopping for paint colors. If someone tells you that you look good in red, they are not really telling you anything. Which red do they mean? Is it intense or muted, light, medium, or dark? You can wear any color; it's the type of color that matters." Giella

Color Principles
"There are three basic rules of color theory that are important to understand for makeup application. As women, we all know these rules and have used them since we first started to shop for clothing, but we never think about applying them to the face.

1. Light colors make things look bigger, and darker colors diminish or make them look smaller. Think about this when you choose a lip color. Dark lip colors look awful on thin lips. It makes the woman look like she has a slit of a mouth, like she's hard or mad.
2. Colors have the inherent ability to absorb or reflect light. All warm colors reflect light. So if you want your skin to look more perfect, or your eyelids not to look crepey, or to reduce discoloration, try a warm color of foundation or a warm shade of eye shadow. The color can be as brilliant as canary yellow or as muted as rusty brown. A warm color, like a warm coral or the colors of fire, draws attention to lips. They appear brighter because they reflect so much light. Cool colors, like the colors of the ocean or forest, or any gray-based colors, absorb light. They are the natural contouring

color tones. One of my pet peeves is when you get a young lady at a makeup counter, who just moved over from handbags, advising you to use a taupe shadow because taupe looks good on everybody. It doesn't look good on everybody. If you have yellow in your skin, it makes you look tired, and it makes deep set eyes look more deep set. Taupe is a contour color. It should go on the bone, but on the lid, it's not your best bet. It works on people with big eyes who want a dramatic look, but it's not a universal color.

3. The final color principle is based on complementary colors on the color wheel. This is how I choose the colors I use. Complementary colors found opposite each other on the color wheel, when mixed together, neutralize each other. Many women have those blue and violet blood vessels that show through the thin skin under the eye, creating dark circles. Opposite blue on the color wheel, you'll find orange, and opposite violet, you'll find yellow. If you mix yellow and orange together, you get a peachy color. Peachy concealers are the best for getting rid of blue-violet shadows. A whitish concealer only gives you a lighter shade of gray. If you look at a baby's skin, and see how translucent it is, it has that pinky-peach hue that's so healthy and gorgeous. That's what you are creating when you use a peachy concealer. It's also a warm color, so it helps get rid of hyperpigmentation. Bobbi Brown came to the realization that all skin is not pink, and she started creating yellow-based products, but for those of us who are yellow, it can make us look sick. That's why I turned to peach. Understanding the concept of complementary colors is very useful in makeup application. For example, red and green are complementary colors. If you put them side by side, they make each other appear brighter and more vibrant. This is called simultaneous contrast. Women always ask me how they can make their brown eyes more exciting. But brown eyes have so many other colors in them: gold, orange, red, green. It's about pulling that color out and making it more exciting. Find the other color that is in there with the brown, and refer to your color wheel for its complementary color. Use that complementary color to line the eye. For example, if you have golden tones in your eye, line it with purple, because that's the opposite of yellow. If there's red, usually on someone with an ethnic background, use a deep green. If there is orange in your eye, use blue. Be careful with purple eyeliner. Make sure it is not too plummy, because this can make you look sick or like you've been crying. Another way to apply complementary colors is to tone down a lipstick shade. If you just put on an orange lipstick and it looks horrible, pick another lipstick or a gloss with a blue or violet base and apply it on top of the orange. It will tone down the orange and make it more comfortable for you to wear. I run into women with a lot of blue-violet pigment in their lips who say that they can't use a bright lip color because everything turns burgundy on them. If you use a coat of gold lipstick first, before your regular lipstick, it will give you that brightness and tone down the blue." Hollis Wright

Beauty School

"If you want to look really beautiful and not like you have a lot of makeup on, go for a monochromatic makeup look. Then you'll see just the features and not the makeup. A lot of times, if you are wearing one color on eyes and another on cheeks and another on lips, you start to look too painted. Experimentation is great when you are really young, and it can be fun as you get older, but be sure to use color to pull out your own features and not to draw attention to the makeup." Bobbe Joy

Color Counsel

"Color theory is a set of principles used to create harmonious color combinations. Color relationships can be visually represented with a color wheel—the color spectrum wrapped onto a circle. For the purposes of color correcting and camouflage, we deal mostly with the Complementary Color Scheme. On the color-wheel spectrum, yellow is the opposite of violet; green is the opposite of red. Using opposites is also how painters tone down bright colors (or neutralize). When applied under foundation as a primer, the corrector colors create a flawless palette. Using opposing colors, you can cover and neutralize areas to help camouflage and create a 'normal' skintone.

"Warm colors reflect light, so they help get rid of darkness like dark circles and hyperpigmentation. Cool colors absorb light, so they create natural contours. Cool contours on the cheeks emphasize high cheekbones. Warm colors along the bone and on the apples of the cheeks will make the cheekbones more prominent. Here's how color theory can be put to use to conceal and camouflage.

Problem

Red, irritated skin caused by acne, broken capillaries, rosacea, microdermabrasion

Solution

Use a yellow or green neutralizer, depending on skintone, to tone down discolorations. Fair skintones should use a yellow product, like Colorescience Yellow Rose of Texas, while darker skintones should use a green product, like Colorescience Mint Condition.

Problem

Yellow, dull skin caused by aging, exhaustion, or sickness

Solution

Use a lavender corrective primer, like Colorescience Snow Leopard.

Problem

Violet skin discolorations such as dark undereye circles, port wine marks, varicose veins

Solution

Use a lavender corrective primer, like Colorescience Snow Leopard.

"Use an orange-peach primer. Begin by applying Colorescience Bye Bye Blues concealer, Per•fekt, or Bombshell Genie and color lightly to the desired area of coverage and blend lightly, smoothing with a sponge. Do not apply heavily."

Diane Ranger

COLORS FOR YOUR UNIQUE COLORING

The Buzz from the Beauty Editor

I've always instinctively rebelled against the warm colors that are supposed to be perfect for my olive skin. First of all, I don't like limitations. Second, warm tones are generally not my favorites. I've always favored cooler colors. Fortunately, the current consensus is that any skintone can wear almost any color. Cooler-toned women no longer need to shun warm colors, and I no longer need to feel guilty about choosing black over brown. What is clear is that choosing colors in the same "temperature" as your skin, whether warm or cool, will make you look more natural, while doing the opposite will produce a more dramatic effect.

Insider Information from the Beauty Bunch

Color Me Cornered

"There have been many theories and systems designed to help women choose the right colors. At one point, I was involved with Color Me Beautiful, but that focused on a teeny-tiny color chart with fabric swatches. It had the opposite effect that it was intended to have; instead of expanding a woman's horizons and allowing her to use more color, it stunted creativity. In Color Me Beautiful, I am a summer, which means that I shouldn't wear black or cool muted colors, but I wear black all the time. But one of the things that you need to remember when discussing makeup colors is that it's not color like you would use to dress yourself or upholster a couch. Makeup colors are sheer washes of color that go over another color that already exists—your skin color. Wardrobe colors are not necessarily the best colors to use on the face. Innately, as human beings, we appreciate these concepts even if we are not consciously aware of them. You are innately attracted to your own best colors, but your mother or friends may have steered you away from them." Hollis Wright

Shopping by Skintone

"There is no hard and fast rule about women with warm skintones wearing warm makeup colors, and women with cool skintones wearing cool colors. Styles change. The more natural you want your makeup to look, the more you coordinate with your skin's undertone. The more dramatic you want to look, the more opposite you go from your skintone. Warm skin looks earthy and natural in bronze lipstick, but at night, for impact, a warm-toned woman can wear cherry-red or magenta. It depends on the effect you want to create. Which feature do you want to draw attention to? That's why I don't like those types of limits. If you tell a cool-toned woman that she can only wear cool colors, then she will never have the advantage of wearing a warm brown and making her eyes appear less crepey, or using peach to make her blue eyes pop." Hollis Wright

Limitless Color

"You don't need to be limited by your skintone. I think every woman should have a range of colors in her makeup wardrobe, from bronze and gold and copper to more fun colors like pinks and purples. Of course, olive skin always looks good in bronze and apricot, and light skin always looks good in pinks and greens, but there are no real rules. I love purple and green on olive skin, for example. Some women have told me that they've always been told to stick to neutrals, but that they are bored with them. If you love color, wear color. Do your neutral makeup as usual and then incorporate just a little bit of bright color. A thin line of blue or green liner inside the eyes gives a nice shot of color without being too much." Meg Thompson

Giella's Color Classifications

"Blondes look best in medium value, medium intensity, and either cool or warm undertones, depending on your skin color. For example, if you want to wear a red, try a red that is not too dark and not too light. It should not have a sharp contrast from your hair and eye color. Blondes can wear any color—pink, brown, coral, rust, plum, or red—it just depends on the shade, depth, and undertone. Colors are really generic.

"If you have dark hair and fair skin, you look best in colors that have depth and have medium to dark intensity. By this, I mean that light (pastels) and muted (khaki, beige, or olive) colors will not be your best choice. You need high contrast because your hair and skin color have a high contrast, so deeper browns, blues, reds, greens, and grays are better for you. For example, a deeper orange would look more like rust or sienna than pumpkin.

"If you have dark hair, dark eyes, and olive skin, you look best in colors that are deeper in value (not light and not muted) and clearer in color (brighter and more vibrant). Examples are midnight navy, ruby red, magenta, indigo violet, mahogany brown, black, and white.

"Most people fall into two of our categories: CPN (Color Profile Neutral) and CPD (Color Profile Dark.) However, there are two other categories: CPL (Color Profile Light) and CPV (Color Profile Vivid.) Here are the descriptions:

CPN: Looks best in medium value color, not too light and not too dark. It's best to choose colors that are earthy, muted, that have a little brown in them. Avoid colors that are very bright or deep.

CPD: Looks best in colors that are deeper in value, not light and not earthy. It's best to choose colors that are clear, sharp, and have a higher contrast with your skin and hair color. Avoid colors that are too muted.

CPL: Looks best in colors that are light to medium in value, not dark. It's best to choose colors that are pastel and have less contrast with hair, eye, and skin color. Avoid colors that are deep and intense.

CPV: Looks best in colors that are brighter in value, not dark. It's best to choose colors that are vibrant, colorful, and contrast with hair, eye, and skin color. Avoid colors that are muted." Giella

Giella's Color Chart

Hair
Light to Dark Blonde,
Strawberry Blonde

Eyes
Hazel, Green, Blue, Brown

Skin
Light to Medium

Grouping
CPN

Hair
Light to Dark Blonde

Eyes
All

Skin
Medium to Dark

Grouping
CPN

Hair
Light Brown to Medium Brown

Eyes
Hazel, Green, Blue, Brown

Skin
Light to Medium

Grouping
CPN

Hair
Light Brown to Medium Brown

Eyes
Hazel, Green, Blue, Brown

Skin
Medium to Dark

Grouping
CPN

Hair
Dark Brown to Black

Eyes
Hazel, Green, Blue, Brown

Skin
Light to Medium

Grouping
CPD

Hair
Dark Brown to Black

Eyes
Hazel, Green, Blue, Brown

Skin
Medium to Dark

Grouping
CPD

Addition / Subtraction

"In theory, the subtractive color processes work by blocking out parts of the spectrum. The idea of subtractive color is to reduce the amount of undesired color reaching the eye. If, for example, you had red skin conditions, you would use a cosmetic color that would let green and blue reach the eye and would absorb the red. In theory, the color additive to do this is cyan (greenish blue). In reality, yellow works most of the time because of the skintone combined with red.

"So in theory, magenta would absorb green. In reality, when you add a skintone, like beige, it will appear gray or sallow, not actually green. Therefore, instead of a bright pink, use a pale pink or lavender to neutralize the sallow skintone. In theory, yellow absorbs blue. In reality, the skin is blue blended with a skintone so apricot or orange will work best. For black or brown, a combination of all three primary colors should block out all light. This is why covering hyperpigmentation is the most difficult. While we use all three colors, we actually take extra steps to achieve this. We start with a blending primer complex to even the skintone. Then, we actually blend a foundation color two shades lighter than the skin. Next, we come back in with the actual skintone color. Finally, we use a deeper skintone to contour and blend. The art of distraction becomes essential here to take the eye away from the discoloration that may or may not be completely concealed." Diane Ranger

Diane Ranger's Additive Secondary/Subtractive Primaries Absorption Chart

Color	Reflects in Theory	Reflects in Reality	Absorbs
Yellow	Red and Green	Apricot/Orange	Blue
Magenta	Red and Blue	Pink/Lavender	Green/Gray
Cyan	Green and Blue	Yellow/Green	Red

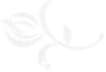

CONCEALING WITH MINERAL AND PERMANENT MAKEUP

The Buzz from the Beauty Editor

When I first started experimenting with mineral makeup, I held on to my cream concealer, convinced that the sheer, featherweight minerals wouldn't conceal everything I wanted to hide. I was wrong. All it took was a little practice, and soon, I was covering everything quickly and invisibly. The following techniques will show you to take cover using mineral makeup.

Scar Strategy

"To camouflage scarring, you should literally 'paint' in the lighter-colored skin. Then even out the edges and blend all the colors together. Colorescience Line Tamer or Mild to Wild can be used to fill in the area that is scarred. Set with finishing powder, and then add loose or pressed minerals. In some cases, a good foundation is all that is needed. Then use the art of distraction. A hairstyle alone can cover the scar area. Another trick is to emphasize other features so that the scar becomes invisible. The secret to applying minerals is layering! You can add as many layers of minerals as you like as long as you keep the layers very sheer. Build color upon color with just a little product at a time. Use Colorescience brushes to detail problem areas. You may 'stipple' hard-to-cover areas with extra pigment. Then set it with a spritzer. Let it dry and then continue to blend an overall color into the rest of the skin." Diane Ranger

Scar Setbacks

"A good candidate for scar camouflage using micropigmentation (permanent cosmetics) is someone who does not tan their skin or who plans to have the procedure done on an area that does not tan, like the stomach. Pigment does not tan. Sun exposure causes pigment to fade. The base pigment for all skintones, except African American skin, is titanium dioxide, which is pure white. So when you are correcting a scar, the colored pigments will fade but the white will never fade. When the other pigments fade, you are sometimes left with a scar that is more obvious than what you started with. There are other methods for camouflaging a scar, so if another method will work for you, I recommend it instead." Kari Boatner

Spritz Solution

"When you are correcting a variety of different skin conditions and colors, it is often necessary to 'camouflage the camouflage.' Using our Achromatherapy Gem Spritzers with a mineral pigment of your choice, you can instantly create a thin spray for an 'airbrush' application that gives the best coverage. Use a drape to protect surrounding areas. To create an airbrush foundation or spray-on bronzer, pour approximately one teaspoon of pigment into about a half bottle of the spritzer and shake. Camouflage the camouflage, spray on a tan or a glow, and add sun protection with one spritz. Use more pigment for more coverage and less pigment for less coverage. If the mineral is 'spitting out,' add more spritzer." Diane Ranger

Camouflage Course

Diane Ranger offers the following techniques for concealing using mineral makeup:

- **Rest and Rock:** to get full coverage on challenging skin, use the "rest and rock" technique. Rest the sponge onto the product and rock onto the skin. Use firm downward pressure to the skin, rocking the hand back and forth so pigment adheres to the skin. Do not move applicator from the initial contact point. Pressed minerals with a sponge give the most intense coverage. These minerals have been micronized multiple times and then "compressed," giving more pigment per square inch.
- **Stipple:** to get full coverage on a targeted area, like a birthmark, age spot, or blemish, use the "stipple" technique with an eye blender brush. Brush concentrated pigment onto the flat side of the brush. Then "stipple"—press the flat side of the brush into the skin with short swift movements—the pigment onto the targeted area.
- **The Hula:** use this technique to camouflage hard-to-cover, detailed fine lines, such as the edges of a tattoo or deep inset lines under the eyes or on the nasolabial fold. Take a straight brow/liner brush and press the end directly into the pigment at a perpendicular angle. Move back and forth without lifting the brush, like a hula dance. Now place the pigmented brush straight onto the specific area to be concealed at a perpendicular angle. Move back and forth without lifting the brush (hula). This should give a lot of coverage in a small area.
- **Overall Blending:** use a blender brush to smooth the outer edges of any area that has been camouflaged. Use featherlike strokes with either a small amount of pigment or even no pigment at all to get smooth, soft finished edges.
- **Press and Pat**: for detailed coverage around the eye, use the sponge that comes with your pressed pigment. Literally press the concealer into the skin and pat it to blend. Pat the sponge onto the pressed or loose pigment and pat gently onto the skin. Do not rub. The idea is to get concentrated pigment in concentrated areas. Rub only if you have applied too much. For blending hard-to-reach areas, use an eye shaper brush. A good example of a hard-to-reach area is the inside corner of the eye. Apply pigment to the eye shaper brush and then use the "press and pat" technique. Diane Ranger

THE PRODUCT FILES

Mineral and Airbrushed Makeup

The Buzz from the Beauty Editor

I am amazed by the powers of mineral and airbrushed makeup. They allow you to achieve entirely different effects than you could with traditional makeup. Once, when I had to strut across a stage in a bathing suit (don't ask), I sprayed Classified Cosmetics ERA Face Spray On Foundation all over my legs to conceal any bumps, bruises, or stretch marks. I have to admit that the skin on my legs looked flawless, and to this day, when I see a celebrity with glowing gams, I wonder how much help she got from a bottle.

What the Pros Choose

Mineral makeup is a favorite among several of our experts, both for the way it looks and for what it does for the skin. As Shan Albert puts it, "I'm an esthetician who never wore foundation because I couldn't find one in which all the ingredients were good for the skin, not just one or two good for the skin and the rest far from good, until I discovered mineral makeup—and now I wouldn't be without it. The foundation I absolutely adore is Colorescience F.A.C.E. Crème de la Crème. It's natural, it covers beautifully, and has an SPF 20—without any chemicals! It makes my skin look flawless—and even with my oily skin, it stays looking great from early morning till late at night." Albert also turns to mineral makeup to hide flaws. She simply applies it with a damp sponge. "It covers everything, is waterproof, and best of all, it's good for the skin," she raves. She has two picks for mineral concealers: Jane Iredale and La Bella Donna. Lilly Rivera's mineral makeup of choice is Mineral Powder Foundation and Mineral Loose Powder, both by Skin Blends. One of the most popular powders on the market, Bare Escentuals Mineral Veil, was also popular with our experts. Two of them, Hara Glick and Galit Strugano, chose it. In the bronzer and blush categories, mineral makeup receives two more votes: one from Shan Albert, for Colorescience Face Colore Bronzer Brush in In the Wild, and the other from Meredith Green, for Pur Minerals in Cherry Blossom. Airbrushed makeup also has a fan in Lilly Rivera. Her favorites: Kett Cosmetics Water Based Foundation and Kett Cosmetics Translucent Powder.

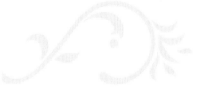

Chapter Five

Enlightening Eye Makeup:
Tools and Techniques for Wink-Worthy Looks

Women have been accentuating their eyes since Cleopatra first brandished a wand of eyeliner. Growing up in an Egyptian family, I was fascinated by one of my mother's only cosmetics: an exotic turquoise vial of kohl. The smudgy, mysterious look it created signaled adulthood to me. Today, eye-makeup options are virtually unlimited, offering endless opportunities for self-expression. Finding a look that accentuates your individual beauty can be tricky, but this chapter offers some tips to help you do it. From choosing an eye-shadow shade that will make your eyes pop to ensuring the shade stays put all day, the tips on these pages will give you something to wink about.

THE *Beauty Bunch* BREAKDOWN

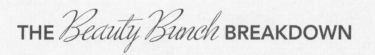

Giella: professional makeup artist and founder of GIELLA Custom Blend Cosmetics.

Wende Zomnir: creative director of Hard Candy Cosmetics and founder/creative director of Urban Decay Cosmetics.

Jeanie Barnett: director of Corporate Communications, Tweezerman.

Bobbe Joy: celebrity makeup artist whose clients include Lucy Liu, Scarlett Johansson, Naomi Watts,

Jennifer Tilly, and Janice Dickinson, she also has a signature line of products, Makeup! Bobbe Joy.

Manana Dzhanimanova: senior eyebrow designer at Frédéric Fekkai.

Anastasia Soare: dubbed the Eyebrow Queen, her work has graced the world's most famous faces, including those of Madonna, Jennifer Lopez, Renee Zellweger, Debra Messing, Oprah Winfrey, Penelope Cruz, and Reese Witherspoon.

Galit Strugano: makeup artist and creator of Girlactik Beauty, a top-selling makeup line.

Stephen Sollitto: sought-after celebrity makeup artist whose clients include Christina Aguilera, Rosario Dawson, Jewel, Erika Christensen, and Tara Reid.

Kari Boatner: permanent-cosmetics pioneer who has developed innovative instruments and artistic procedures for the application of permanent makeup.

Diane Gardner: Hollywood hairstylist, colorist, and makeup artist known as the Makeover Specialist.

Terri Apanasewicz: celebrity makeup artist with L.A.'s Cloutier Agency whose clients have included Michael Michele, Jeri Ryan, Kristin Davis, Toni Braxton, and Reba McEntire.

Lilly Rivera: celebrated makeup artist at the prestigious Dominique Salon in the Hotel Pierre, New York City.

Debra Macki: a top Boston-based makeup artist and the founder of Debra Macki Cosmetics.

THE BEST OF THE BASICS

The Buzz from the Beauty Editor

Eye makeup is the only makeup I consider optional. I have large, dark eyes and full lashes, so during the day, I skip eye makeup entirely. At night, I like to be more adventurous, using shimmery shadows to brighten my perpetually dark eye area, and liquid liner (always black) to elongate my round eyes. And when I go out, I want to make sure that it lasts. That's why the stay-put tips that follow are so important.

Insider Information from the Beauty Bunch

Prime Time

The pros, including Giella and Wende Zomnir, recommend using a primer under your shadow to make it last. "You'll still look fresh at the end of the day," raves Zomnir, who recommends Urban Decay Primer Potion. Giella agrees: "A lot of women complain that they can't keep their shadow on for long, and that it creases by midday, but they don't realize that you need to use a shadow base. The right base can keep eye shadow on for twelve hours, and it lightens the eyelid so that your regular skin color doesn't show through when you use a pale shade of eye shadow. The skin on your eyelid is actually darker than the skin under your eye."

Long-Lasting Looks

"For extra long–lasting eye makeup, use your shadow wet. Not liquid-y—more like a paste. And set your eye pencil with a similar-colored shadow dabbed on top with a flat, stiff brush." Wende Zomnir

Major Mistakes

"One of the biggest makeup mistakes that women make is to put eyeliner on the bottom so that it goes all the way in, to the corner of the eye. It should only be one-third to one-half of the way in. Otherwise, you close your eye up completely and it looks like you have these two holes in your head. And don't skip liner on the bottom. It won't accentuate dark circles if you've done the rest of your makeup correctly. Eyeliner on the bottom draws attention to the eye itself, so that you don't notice the dark circles. Another mistake is not curling lashes, and not applying mascara to the bottom lashes. You have lashes there, so you should use mascara on those lashes or it looks unbalanced." Bobbe Joy

ENCHANTING EYELINERS

The Buzz from the Beauty Editor

I am a huge fan of eyeliner. I love how instantly transforming it can be—and how dramatic. In addition to my passion for black liquid liners, I also love glittery eyeliners. They add sparkle and subtle definition while bringing eyes to life, and they're much more subtle than they sound. Makeup artists often line the inside of the eyes with white liners to brighten them and make them appear open, and I've adapted this trick to my darker skintone. I use a light beige liner instead of a white one to get the same effect in a more subtle way.

Insider Information from the Beauty Bunch

Divine Define

"To really define eyes without a heavy look, line the upper inner lid of your eyes. It's freaky at first, but addictive once you try it." Wende Zomnir

Thin Line

"Pull lid tight with finger—dip a thin brush in liquid liner and line in the groove between lashes and lid. This will get a very thin, even line. Try cake liners, which enable you to decide the consistency of your liner. Cake liners are mixed with water, and you can judge how strong the color is by testing on your hand before applying to your eyes." Giella

Liquid or Pencil

"Liquid is harder to apply, but offers more geometric definition. It takes practice and a steady hand to apply it well. Pencil is easier and more versatile." Terri Apanasewicz

Aging Eyeliner

"The number-one thing women do that makes them look older is [the way they apply their] eyeliner. Absolutely. They are wearing it completely around the entire eyeball. All the young starlets like Britney Spears, the young girls that want to look older, do it, and they are the perfect example of what not to do. Twenty-four is the turning point, where if you wear that kind of makeup you look old and tired. It's way too heavy of a makeup and makes eyes look heavy and tired. The way to avoid this is to line the top lid, along the lash line, beginning where the hair starts and stopping where it ends, with pencil or liquid. And here's where you clean it up and make it not so heavy. On the bottom, you start in the center of the eye and take an eye pencil (not liquid liner, which is too harsh) and just start smudging between the hairs on the bottom, between eyelashes, very lightly. Go to where the hair stops and leave the rest of the eye free of eyeliner. If you look in the mirror, you'll see that's a whole quarter-inch on the outside and inside corner that's left without liner. It opens the eye, and it looks more almond-shaped and bright. Eyeliner all the way around makes eyes look smaller, and it's really aging, especially if you are forty-plus and your eyes are drooping. You get all the definition and drama, but the eyes look open. To get a smoky effect, use a brush and go over the top of the liner to soften it." Diane Gardner

PERFECTLY GROOMED BROWS

The Buzz from the Beauty Editor
I have dark, moderately thick eyebrows, so grooming is essential. When my brows are groomed, my eyes appear brighter, cleaner, and more awake. Since my eyebrows are curly, I fill in any gaps with pencil or powder. And when I apply a face mask, I smooth some on my brows to straighten them out. It really seems to work.

Insider Information from the Beauty Bunch

Symmetrical Brows
"The most important thing is for your brows to be symmetrical, to keep your face symmetrical. Especially with dark hair, which shows every shape." Manana Dzhanimanova

Shaping Up
"I prefer both [waxing and tweezing]: waxing to remove all hairs, including the fine hairs that cannot be plucked out, and tweezing for precision shaping right after waxing. The best way to determine the ultimate shape for you is to stand in front of a mirror with a pencil, and hold it upright from the middle of your nostril straight up—this is where your brow should start. Then hold the pencil vertically from the tip of your nose above your iris. This is where the highest point of your brow arch should be. Lastly, hold the pencil from the corner of your nose to the corner of your eye; this is where the brow should end. After establishing the beginning and end of your brow, tweeze with caution in order to achieve the best shape. Use slant-tip tweezers, and hold the skin down gently while carefully removing one hair at a time. Slant tips are the best; they don't pinch the skin and will not break the hairs. Brows should be professionally shaped once a month; you can tweeze a few stray hairs every week. To keep brows in place, use a brow gel like Anastasia Beverly Hills Tinted Brow Gel. It is flake-free and super gentle on the skin." Anastasia Soare

Clean Shape
"I think waxing is cleaner. You should have your brows professionally shaped every three to four weeks." Manana Dzhanimanova

Filling in the Gap
"The most common mistake women make is over-tweezing. The best remedy is brow powder to fill in during the growth process. Use a good powder in a color close to your natural hair, and an angled brush. [Note: Anastasia recommends stencils to help with shaping.] Fill in daily in order to give the appearance of brows, and once they have grown in, you can start arching and shaping using tweezers." Anastasia Soare

Curly Brows
"Curly eyebrows have to be trimmed. It helps a lot. I brush them up and trim them. You should also pencil in bald spots. I prefer pencil to powder because it

lasts longer. First, let them grow so you can see what they look like. In a few months, you will know if you have hair there. Sometimes, women will pull out the long ones and then they'll have bald patches." Manana Dzhanimanova

Perfect Pairs?

"Brows are never exactly alike. I try to make them as symmetrical as possible using powder and pencil." Anastasia Soare

Pain Pill

"Take Advil before a tweezing appointment to ease the discomfort." Manana Dzhanimanova

Plucking Pointers

"Do keep brows more natural. There is always room for extra plucking later. Don't try to copy an eyebrow style out of a magazine. It won't come out exactly as it looks in the magazine and probably won't be the best shape for you. Do tell your eyebrow artist if you are using Accutane or Retin-A. [Note: Waxing skin that is being treated with Retin-A or Accutane can lead to discomfort, burning, and peeling.] Do use brow gel as a daily conditioner for optimal hair growth." Anastasia Soare

Top Tweezers

"I like Tweezerman tweezers, the ones with the pointy tip, not the slanted tip." Manana Dzhanimanova

Painless Plucking

"Avoid waxing around your menstrual period, or when your heart rate is up. For eliminating redness, visit a professional who uses wax for sensitive skins (liposoluble or Azulene wax). This will help minimize redness and pain. Also use pre- and post-tweeze creams." Anastasia Soare

Gel or Tell

"I am not a fan of eyebrow gel. It made my brows fall out. If you trim them, they'll stay in place." Manana Dzhanimanova

Brow Benefits

Reshaping brows is the "best makeover for a mature woman. It works wonders on someone who can't wear eye makeup because of excessive wrinkles. Brows that are thin and light only draw more attention to wrinkles. Balance the brows. If brows droop, tweeze away the drooping end and fill in higher brows with pencil. Accent the browbone with matte highlighter. Well-groomed and defined brows can make someone look ten years younger." Debra Macki

Thicker Is Better

"I love thick eyebrows. I've always liked thick eyebrows. They're always in style. I think you can shape them well. They're more beautiful and flattering. The impression is so different when you have fuller eyebrows. Thin eyebrows give you more age. Some people don't have thick eyebrows, and you have to work with whatever you have. Keep them as full as possible; full but groomed looks younger." Manana Dzhanimanova

Tweeze Tips

"Ease the tweeze by taking a shower or placing a hot washcloth over your brow. This opens pores. Never use an ice cube or freeze the tweezer. This closes pores and makes it harder to pull hair. Skip creams and moisturizers too—they can make the tweezers slippery. Study the hair you are about to tweeze and determine the direction in which it grows. For example, above and below the nose, it grows vertically; above the eye and on the cheek, it grows horizontally. There are exceptions, so look closely at your own hair before you begin.

"Choose your tool. A slant tweezer is ideal for general tweezing and for reaching tiny hairs. A point tweezer is extremely accurate and preferred by most professionals. It can remove any hair, including ingrown hairs. A pointed slant is a combination of the point and slant tweezers. A body tweezer is ideal for chin-, leg-, and bikini-area use. It grabs difficult-to-reach coarse hairs and can be used to remove stubble and ingrown hairs.

"Next, using an eyebrow brush, brush hair in the direction of hair growth. Isolate the hair you are about to tweeze. Always tweeze in the direction of the hair growth. Pull one hair out at a time. Pull gently and smoothly—don't yank! Post-plucking, you'll want to follow-up with an astringent. It will clean and close pores. After tweezing ingrown hairs, clean the area with hydrogen peroxide. Wait at least a half hour before applying creams or moisturizers." Jeanie Barnett

Uneven Brows

"Many people, without realizing it, lift one brow more than the other while talking. Over time, the one eye muscle is much stronger and higher. Try to pay attention to which eyebrow you lift while talking and then exercise the other. Lift the weaker eyebrow several hundred times during the day to strengthen the muscle. It's important to make a consistent effort for at least six months. Also, have a professional analyze your brows and perhaps a shaping will help even your brows a little." Giella

Tweeze in Moderation

"Be careful: if you tweeze a lot, it may take a long time to grow back." Manana Dzhanimanova

Getting Rid of Grays

"Plucking gray hairs is not a good idea because it will cause holes in your brow. Instead, cover them up by running some tinted brow gel through them." Giella

Tweezer Touch-Ups

"I have clients who don't touch [their brows between appointments] and those who love to touch. Don't go too close to the shape. Just tweeze the very low ones or a stray hair. With dark hair, it's hard to wait for three weeks, so just tweeze the low ones." Manana Dzhanimanova

Shaping Brows

"Try to find an eyebrow shape you like in a magazine, one that will compliment your face. Take it to a professional so that they can do it for you and teach you at the same time. I recommend a professional because trimming, tweezing, and measuring are involved. Remember brows are not twins; they are sisters. So don't panic if they are slightly off. There are a few ways to shape brows: tweezing, threading, waxing, and shaving. I recommend tweezing or threading. However, threading is hard to find, and may not be as precise.

"I do not recommend waxing because it's harsh on your skin and may cause a burning effect and broken capillaries. It may be quicker but it usually results in more hairs being ripped off than you wanted. It's also difficult to get precise with hot wax because it spreads so quickly. I've seen some experts do a great job at waxing, but there are some areas where waxing just doesn't work; tweezers are more precise. Shaving is the quickest and least painful but it can cause cuts and scarring, and usually leaves stubble. Thus, tweezing is the way to go! My favorite tweezers are Mehaz by Rubis. They come in slanted and pointed tips. They are precise and effective, and so lightweight. The slant is great

for grown hair. The pointed is great for stubble and ingrown hairs." Giella

Above the Brow
"Some people like [removing hair above the brow] and some don't. If it's shaped nicely, you don't have to wax. You can trim or shape a few hairs. It grows the same as the rest of your eyebrow. But if you don't know what you're doing, you can ruin everything. My clients don't touch above the brow." Manana Dzhanimanova

Brow Maintenance
"It's best to have your brows maintained every month so that you do not have to start from scratch every time. If you are upkeeping them yourself, look at them once a week and pull the little hairs that are growing in. Looking at your brows every day can usually lead to trouble. People have a tendency to take out the wrong hair and go back and forth until it's even, and wind up with thinner and thinner brows. However, some people are blessed with very full brows and might need to check three to four times a week. Don't overwax or tweeze, because your brows might not grow back in." Giella

Permanently Perfect Brows Using Micropigmentation
"I start by drawing a brow on. It takes me forty-five minutes to draw on eyebrows that are symmetrical, that match each other. I measure each part of the brow. There are three steps to creating beautiful brows. The first is picking the color. I choose a neutral color and smear it between the brows, thinly enough so that you can see the natural skintone through it. A neutral color consists of fifty-percent cool pigment and fifty-percent warm pigment; they cancel each other out. Then I examine the color. I want it to blend; I don't want anything to stand out.

Does it look cool or warm, blue or orange? If I see orange, it means that the client has warm skin; blue indicates cool skin. If the skin is warm, I pick a cool color, because the warmth in the skin cancels out the cool in the pigment and makes it neutral.

"I don't do single-color brows because they are not natural. Very rarely do you see someone with one solid color in their brows, unless their hair is jet black. Blondes, for example, have some blonde and some brown. If you incorporate more than one color, you get a natural, wispy look. The second step is determining the width, and the third is determining how close to make the hair strokes. For softer eyebrows, you should use wide strokes; for more dense eyebrows, more strokes. Then I use simulated hair strokes to draw on the brow." Kari Boatner

Individual Shape
"Everyone has a different shape. You can't give everyone the same shape. Everyone likes a nice arch. Women don't like round brows, even if they have long faces. When I see a face, if it's strong, I do an arch but a soft arch. Not too archy. If they have a soft look, then I do a bigger arch to look sexy. I know right away what a client needs. For dark brows or dark coloring, go for less of an arch, or it looks too severe. But for a blonde, I can go to archier. If they know what they want, I will take their input before I start." Manana Dzhanimanova

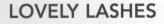

LOVELY LASHES

The Buzz from the Beauty Editor

My lashes are naturally long, full, and dark, but I love to play them up with mascara, particularly in the evening. One of my favorite tricks is to add very subtle color to my dark eyes with a colored mascara in a shade like midnight blue, eggplant, or teal. The effect is striking without being obvious, and it really wakes up tired eyes. And to avoid the spiky, spidery look, I use a metal lash separator to comb through my lashes right after applying mascara. But because my lashes are long and curly, I never thought I needed to curl my lashes until a close girlfriend (who's a professional) permed them for me. It changed my life. I couldn't stop staring at my eyes. Suddenly, my eyes seemed more open and my lashes longer than ever—without mascara. Now I'm hooked. I get my lashes permed whenever I can, and in between, I use an eyelash curler. *[Note: Don't try perming your eyelashes at home. Go to a reputable salon or spa for this service.]*

Insider Information from the Beauty Bunch

Lower Lashes

Should mascara be applied to the lower lashes? "It all depends on what type of look you are trying to achieve. If you are doing an evening or smoky or dramatic eye with eyeliner on the top and bottom, it's more effective to wear mascara on both the top and bottom. If you are wearing a very natural eye make-up, you might want to use more mascara on top of your lashes and then lightly coat the tips of the lashes underneath. If you have a tendency to have darker circles under your eyes, have small eyes, or are very oily around the eye area, it's best to leave it very clean and light under the eyes and concentrate on lining and defining the top of your eyes. However, if a water-resistant mascara is applied lightly, it can work." Giella

Budget Buy

Women should splurge on eye cream, but save on mascara, according to celebrity makeup artist Terri Apanasewicz.

Mascara Maneuver

"Most women, when they apply mascara, don't really roll it on underneath the base of the lash, but you really should do that. Tilt your head back and keep rolling the brush up and under, right at the lashline. Your lashes will look so much thicker. For a nice dramatic effect, dab some eyeliner between your upper lashes." Giella

Ageless Eyes

"If your eyelashes don't curl anymore, mascara and an eyelash curler, used skillfully, will open up the eyes for a youthful appearance. If your eyes are droopy, smudge liner thickly at outer upper corner of eyes and use mascara on outer upper lashes only." Debra Macki

Long-Lasting Lashes

"For gorgeous, natural-looking lashes, I apply long-wearing lash extensions, lash by lash. The result is fuller, longer, more fabulous lashes. The extensions are undetectable to the naked eye, and last about two months or until your own lashes grow out. There is no need for additional mascara since the lash line is designed to be fuller and the lashes longer. They're

medium-toned matte color all over lid. Apply liner to lashline, making it thicker at the outer third of the eye. Very little or no eyeliner on bottom lashline. Light coat of mascara on top lashes. Avoid frosted or shimmery eye colors."

Smoky Stare
"Try two tones of a dark color—it doesn't have to be black and gray. Apply the lighter color all over the lid and then, with the darker of the two, apply near the lashline and out to the corner in a "V" shape. Blend out and up. On the bottom, use the darkest color near the lashline on the outside third of the eye and use the lighter one across the whole length of the bottom and blend." Terri Apanasewicz

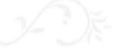

APPLY YOURSELF

The Buzz from the Beauty Editor
Application is everything. A bold, brazen color that looks virtually unwearable can be stunning if the application is sheer. That's why it's essential to try a color before you dismiss it; colors can look dramatically different on your face than they do in the pot.

Insider Information from the Beauty Bunch

Bright Eyes
"Try a light, iridescent color all over lids for a vibrant look." Terri Apanasewicz

Intense Color
"Dab your shadow on when you apply it," Galit Strugano advises, "because then the color is solid rather then blended on the eye. It looks more intense." Bobbe Joy agrees: "For a soft natural eye shadow look, brush color onto the lid, but for more intensity, lay it on instead of brushing it on. To apply color in the crease, use a windshield-wiper motion, back and forth, to blend."

THE PRODUCT FILES

Powder Eye Shadows

The Buzz from the Beauty Editor
I'm not a big eye-shadow person. Usually, I reserve eye makeup for evening, when my black liquid liner and a couple coats of mascara do the trick. If I'm ambitious, I will apply a single shade, usually a pale, shimmery neutral, to my entire lid. I prefer to apply shadow with brushes rather than those dated sponge applicators. The application is smoother, easier, and more even; there's no tugging. Smashbox makes some great shadow brushes. Get "bedroom eyes" by applying a soft, shimmery golden shade to the entire lid up to the brow, and a medium brown in the crease. My favorites are POP Beauty Eye Cake in Brown Eyes, $19, Smashbox Eyelights Palette in Smashing Beam, $32, and Face Stockholm Pearl Eyeshadow in #29, $16.

What the Pros Choose

The pros have definitive—and different—picks for powder eye shadow. Three experts, Meredith Green, Lilly Rivera, and Mala Elhassan, pick MAC shadows—with the matte formulas specifically mentioned. A few shades singled out are Surreal (Elhassan), and Vex, Shroom, Swiss Chocolate, and Texture (all favorites of Rivera). Christian Dior (Julie Hewett) and Make Up For Ever (Galit Strugano) are both chosen for their intense pigments. Danielle Browning loves all the different shades of Pop Eye Cakes. "You can really control the intensity of the color, and the shimmer is subtle and great!" she raves. Debra Macki chooses her own shadow in Honeymoon while Wende Zomnir singles out Urban Decay's Midnight Cowboy Rides Again. Meg Thompson favors NARS Duo Eyeshadow in Key Largo and Becca Loose Shimmer Powder in Odette. Other favorites include Aveda Petal Essence in Spark (Shauna Raisch), Chanel (June Jacobs), Stila in Rain (Dee DeLuca-Mattos), and Tina Earnshaw (Hara Glick).

Cream Eye Shadows

The Buzz from the Beauty Editor

I love cream eye shadows, but they are really only practical, in my opinion, if you are going for a sheer wash of color over the entire lid. They are not as convenient if you are going to use two or three shades, as they typically don't blend well. However, for my favorite look, a liquid liner paired with a quick swipe of shimmery shadow, cream formulas work beautifully. Cream shadows virtually scream for a shadow primer to lock color in place and prevent creasing. It's an extra step, but it's worth it for long-lasting color. My favorites are NARS Cream Eyeshadow in Klondike, $18, and Almay Bright Eyes Color Cream Shadow in Golden Gleam, $5.

What the Pros Choose

Dee DeLuca-Mattos chooses Chanel, while Shan Albert chooses Colorescience Smudge It Eye Shadow (it "goes on like a cream and dries to a powder so it stays put") and Wende Zomnir picks Urban Decay Liquid Liner in Crash. Other picks include Delux Beauty Cream Powder Shadow (Julie Hewett), Aveda Uruku Eye Accent in Yuca (Shauna Raisch), NARS Corfu (Meg Thompson), Benefit (Hara Glick), Origins (June Jacobs), and Stila (Meredith Green).

Eyeliners

The Buzz from the Beauty Editor

I hardly ever wear pencil liners—I prefer the drama, wear, and smooth application of liquid liners. I find liner brushes easier to use than the currently popular felt-tipped pens, but they are increasingly harder to come by. A lot of women are intimidated by liquid liners, but I think they're indispensable. All you need is a steady hand, which you can achieve by resting your elbow on something stable, and a little patience. Use short, feathery strokes rather than attempting one quick swipe across, and wait a moment for it to dry. Once it sets, it will last longer than pencils without smudging or smearing. My favorites are L'Oreal Lineur Intense Defining Liquid Liner, $7, and Anna Sui Liquid Eye Liner, $19.

What the Pros Choose

Three of our pros cite MAC as their liner of choice: Hara Glick loves MAC Kohl liners; Meg Thompson uses MAC Eye Kohl in Teddy; and Lilly Rivera chooses MAC Crème Liner in Black. Wende Zomnir picks Hard Candy Glitter Eye in Cyber; Galit Strugano chooses Girlactik Beauty Sparkle Eye Liner Set; and Debra Macki chooses her own eye pencil in Suede. Danielle Browning chooses Trish McEvoy's Gel Eyeliner: "It goes on like a powder eyeliner but stays in place!" Julie Hewett chooses Guerlain; June Jacobs picks Laura Mercier; Shauna Raisch loves Aveda Petal Essence Eye Definer in Lily; and Dee DeLuca-Mattos loves Chanel. Two budget-friendly options: Meredith Green's choice of Maybelline eyeliners, and Wet 'n' Wild liquid liners, favored by Mala Elhassan.

Mascara (Dramatic)

The Buzz from the Beauty Editor

Mascara is perhaps the most controversial product: no matter what they do, cosmetic companies can't seem to hit on one formula that makes every woman happy. I prefer a thick brush and an intense product that builds thickness and length in one quick step. When I want extra drama, I dust some face powder onto my lashes with a powder puff before applying mascara. It thickens and creates a lush look that's second only to false lashes. My favorites are L'Oreal Voluminous Mascara, $7, Fresh Supernova Mascara, $25, and Lancôme Definicils High Definition Mascara, $21.

What the Pros Choose

Since dramatic is not a quantifiable term, it means different things to different women. For Julie Hewett and Debra Luftman, dramatic lashes call for Lancôme Definicils. For June Jacobs, Lancôme Intencils produces the most dramatic fringe. Galit Strugano and Meg Thompson both choose MAC, with Strugano specifying Splashproof Lash and Thompson singling out Pro Lash. Shauna Raisch and Lilly Rivera both choose Blinc Kiss Me Mascara, and Rivera raves about its benefits: "For smudgeproof, water-resistant mascara, I use Blinc. I begin with the Blinc Heated Lash Curler, which instantly curls your lashes with gentle heat, and then follow with Blinc mascara. I start at the base, apply one coat, and then I move on to the next eye, apply one coat, and move back to add additional coats. It sets in one minute. After that, there is no need for additional coats. Eyes looks great! It does not run or smudge, and gives you fuller, longer lashes. It is removed with water and gentle pressure only; you don't need makeup remover. It's great for sensitive eyes." And what could be more dramatic than a little glitter? Maybe that's why Wende Zomnir picks Hard Candy Glitter Lash Freak. Other picks include Yves Saint Laurent (Mala Elhassan), Christian Dior LongOptic (Dee DeLuca-Mattos), Prescriptives (Meredith Green), Clarins (Linda Deslauriers), and, of course, the very popular Maybelline Great Lash (another pick from Meredith Green).

Mascara (Natural)

The Buzz from the Beauty Editor

Everyone's definition of "natural" is different. To me, a natural mascara is a quick, daytime, out-the-door formula—when I want a polished look without the drama I require at night. I always dab the tip of the mascara wand— where excess mascara tends to collect—onto a tissue before applying it to my lashes to prevent clumping and splattering. My favorites are Almay One Coat Thickening Mascara, $6, and Blinc Kiss Me Mascara, $24.

What the Pros Choose

Though there are no definitive winners in this category, there are a couple of favorites. Hara Glick and Meg Thompson love Shu Uemura. Dee DeLuca-Mattos chooses Maybelline Great Lash, while Julie Hewett prefers Maybelline Lash Discovery. Wende Zomnir chooses Urban Decay Skyscraper Mascara; Meredith Green picks Lamas Lash Masque; Shauna Raisch likes Aveda Mosscara in Black Forest; Mala Elhassan picks Lancôme; June Jacobs loves Lancôme Definicils; and Danielle Browning picks Christian Dior Show. To Shan Albert, "natural" means all-natural ingredients. She thinks Colorescience Thick & Curly Mascara is "amazing," and she offers this tip: "Back in the early sixties, we used to melt mustache wax and brush it on to build incredibly long lashes. We used the wax in place of false lashes, and this mascara allows me to build practically the same results. I apply many thin coats both under and on top of the lashes. With each successive coat, I make the tips longer. I haven't been able to do this with any other mascara, but the trick is to apply thin coats."

Chapter Six

Luscious Lip Makeup:
Play Up Your Pucker with the Top Tips for Your Lips

My very first lip product was a tube of Bonne Bell Strawberry Lip Smacker that made me the envy of all the girls in the fourth grade. And though I've since graduated to more sophisticated lip glosses, I still can't resist yummy flavor and cute packaging. For most of us, lipstick marked our first foray into the grown-up world of cosmetics. It is the first cosmetic we try, and for many, it's the one indispensable part of our beauty routine. I am obsessed with lipstick. I never leave the house without it. More than any other cosmetic, a lipstick has the power to enliven and transform, to whisper or shout.

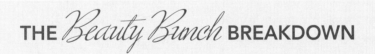

THE Beauty Bunch BREAKDOWN

Jan Marini: skin-care authority and founder of Jan Marini Skin Research.

Michelle Ornstein: owner/founder of Enessa Wellness Spa and its accompanying aromatherapeutic skin-care line.

John Ivey, MD: celebrity cosmetic dentist practicing in Beverly Hills who is known as the Smile Maker.

Debra Macki: a top Boston-based makeup artist and the founder of Debra Macki Cosmetics.

Peter Lamas: founder and chairman of Lamas Beauty International, a rapidly growing, well-respected natural beauty product manufacturer.

Giella: professional makeup artist and founder of GIELLA Custom Blend Cosmetics.

Bobbe Joy: celebrity makeup artist whose clients include Lucy Liu, Scarlett Johansson, Naomi Watts, Jennifer Tilly, and Janice Dickinson, she also has a signature line of products, Makeup! Bobbe Joy.

Diane Gardner: Hollywood hairstylist, colorist, and makeup artist known as the Makeover Specialist.

Stephen Sollitto: sought-after celebrity makeup artist whose clients include Christina Aguilera, Rosario Dawson, Jewel, Erika Christensen, and Tara Reid.

Wende Zomnir: creative director of Hard Candy Cosmetics and founder/creative director of Urban Decay Cosmetics.

Meg Thompson: Hollywood makeup artist and co-owner and founder of Madge Cosmetics.

Kari Boatner: permanent-cosmetics pioneer who has developed innovative instruments and artistic procedures for the application of permanent make-up.

Julie Hewett: top movie-makeup artist for films such as *Pearl Harbor*, *American Beauty*, *Spiderman*, and *Ocean's 11* and *Ocean's 12*, and creator of a bestselling eponymous makeup line.

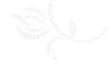

SMILE REMEDIES

The Buzz from the Beauty Editor

I tend to chew on my lips when I am concentrating, so they are perpetually dry. This makes it almost impossible to wear stains or long-wearing lipsticks, which only make dry lips look drier. That's why I make sure to gently exfoliate my lips whenever I can. I find the best way to do this is to use a very warm washcloth in the shower, and gently buff the chapped skin away.

Insider Information from the Beauty Bunch

Rx for Dry Lips

"At night, wipe off your lipstick, then take a wet washcloth and rub it over your lips really vigorously, until they are like satin. Then continue with your skin-care routine, and rub every single thing you put on your face into your lips as well, including AHAs. Then apply a really gooey product, the kind that doesn't sink into the skin, to your lips, and leave on overnight. I like Vaseline, Janet Sartin Superfatted Cream, and Elizabeth Arden Eight Hour Cream. Your lips will have that wonderful occlusive coating all night long, and the next day you will have unbelievably soft lips." Jan Marini

Rosy Glow

"Put a drop of Enessa Aromatherapy Rose Oil on your lips and the corners of your mouth to prevent cracked skin before putting on lipstick and after taking it off." Michelle Ornstein

Smile File

"Avoid or limit foods and beverages that stain teeth, brush the tongue to help eliminate bad breath, and visit your dentist to see if you are a good candidate for professional bleaching and teeth veneers." John Ivey, MD

APPLICATION ADVICE

The Buzz from the Beauty Editor

I always make sure to dab any moisture from my lips before applying lipstick, so it goes on more smoothly. A little dryness actually helps lipstick stick; color won't adhere to lips that are too smooth and slippery.

Insider Information from the Beauty Bunch

Banish Bleeding

"Line lips, avoid gloss, use matte formulas, and set with powder." Debra Macki

Essential Beauty

"A great lipstick [is the one essential]. Every woman looks sexier when her lips are pretty." Peter Lamas

Staying Power

"I have a foolproof secret to keeping lipstick on and keeping it from bleeding. You start by applying foundation over your lips with a sponge. Then take Benefit De Groovie, which is similar to mortician's wax, and pat it around the lip line. Then take face powder and press it over the top and put on lipliner and lipstick, or just lipstick. If you use lipliner, apply lipstick to the edge of the lipliner. If you want, you can apply lip gloss on top and it will not bleed." Jan Marini

Plump Your Pout

"A little white highlighter or powder in the center of your lips, or a dab of gloss, will make them look fuller. Some people say that women over forty shouldn't wear shimmer, but I think that depends. A color with some sheen can be more flattering than a totally matte shade." Giella

Line Errors

"One mistake that many women make is lining their lips inside their natural lipline. If you apply your lipliner properly, your lips will look twice as full." Bobbe Joy

Show-Off Shine

"I like to apply lip gloss over lipstick—it gives a fuller, sexier look." Peter Lamas

Fine Line

"I don't use lipliner on many clients, because as lipstick fades and lipliner stays, they get that ring around the lip. Use lip pencil only [if you don't have a] defined lip. But I do recommend lip pencil for special events and photography. You need more definition for it to show up in a photograph, whether it's a model's photo shoot or a wedding." Diane Gardner

Sheerly Fabulous

"One thing I do on practically everyone I work with is that I take a little Kiehl's lip balm and some lipstick, whatever color I want, and I make a sheer application of it to the lips. It's pretty, not caked on, it keeps lips healthy, and when it dries out, there's a little stain left behind and you can just reapply the lip balm." Stephen Sollitto

Gloss for Good

"For a long-lasting glossy lip, try a double-ended product like Hard Candy Stain & Shine—it stains your lips first, and then adds a coat of pretty gloss." Wende Zomnir

Modern Lips

"Today, the look of lipstick is very sheer, with very little pigmentation. There's more gloss and less pigment. So if you take a shade like a Miami coral—that horrible shade that a lot of women wear—and put it in a gloss, like Chanel Sirop, it looks great on almost everybody." Diane Gardner

Blot and Smooch

"You can make lipstick last longer—even through kissing—by blotting it with powder after application." Peter Lamas

MADE-FOR-YOU SHADES

The Buzz from the Beauty Editor

If you ask my sister what shade of lipstick she's wearing, you will never get a straight answer. She always mixes several shades together until she gets the desired effect. I am usually more straightforward, although I am trying to be more creative. I like a variety of lip colors, from pinks to reds to the occasional neutral, but I always avoid overly pale, frosty glosses, which make my skin look ashy. I recommend avoiding them no matter what your skintone. They are rarely flattering.

Insider Information from the Beauty Bunch

Rut-Busting

"Sticking with a lip color for twenty years ages you." Debra Macki

Neutral Territory

"When choosing a neutral lipstick, pick five shades that you think might look good on you, line them up on the counter, and then apply them to your hand in the same order as they are on the counter, so you don't get mixed up. They will look so different on your skin. Narrow it down to two, and then try them on your lips to see which shade looks best. Go for a neutral with some pink in it. It's more natural and flattering, not brown or muddy. Stila Jane is a great neutral that looks good on everyone." Meg Thompson

Shade Selection

"Pick a shade of lip color based on your skintone. It needs to be in the same colorway as the rest of your makeup. Once you decide you want to do a peachy makeup look, for example, you need to know whether you want peachy gold or peachy pink or peachy bronze, based on your skintone. After that, depending on how much color you need, you pick a gradation from light to dark. A lot of times it's hit and miss until you find the right shade, the shade that will give you sexy lips." Bobbe Joy

Mix or Match

"I don't think there are any steadfast rules about matching lipstick to an outfit, but I've always liked continuity. Use your own judgment. If you're wearing a red dress, you probably don't want to wear burgundy lipstick. You may not pick a perfect-matched red, but you don't want something that

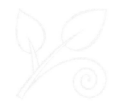

totally clashes, either. I probably wouldn't pick a bubblegum pink, but they might do that at the Prada show next season and pull it off. So I don't think that taking an outfit into account is a bad idea; it's a pretty good formula." Stephen Sollitto

Match Mate
"I like to match lip color to clothes color. A bright red dress will look even hotter if the lip color is equally red." Peter Lamas

Lush Lips
"Many micropigmentation technicians will do a lip line, but I won't. I want to look good for my husband, and I know when I wake up in the morning, if I have this dark line around my mouth, it's going to look awful. So I do either a complete lip fill or a line and shade, where the color starts out darker on the lip line and then is feathered into the inside of the lips, getting lighter, like natural lip color. The result is a fresh, youthful lip color, like a baby's. I pick the shade based on the natural lip color, but if lips are faded I'll go for a little more color, since lips are an accent. I use warm colors on cool-toned women and cool colors on warm-toned women because the skin's natural and opposing pigment will neutralize the color." Kari Boatner

Salvaging a Scary Shade
"If you have a shade of lipstick that's too bright or doesn't work for some reason, tone it down with a colored gloss. This creates the most beautiful effect. I love fuchsia lipstick with apricot gloss, or magenta lipstick with a soft brown gloss." Meg Thompson

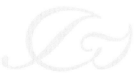

RED REDUX

The Buzz from the Beauty Editor
Red is my best color, and one of my favorites. I especially love red lipstick, because it is so dramatic and flattering, but unfortunately, my husband is not a fan, so I wear it only occasionally. The rest of the time, I content myself with pinks and the occasional pinkish-beige, because I think rosy tones add warmth and softness to a complexion.

Insider Information from the Beauty Bunch

Picking the Perfect Red
"It all depends on your hair, eye, and skin color. If you are blonde, strawberry blonde, or light brown with fair complexion and have blue, hazel, green, or brown eyes, you would fall into a category that would be a CPN. A CPN does not have a sharp contrast between their hair, eye, and skin color. Therefore, the best red for a CPN would be a medium-value red (not too dark and not too light) with medium intensity. It would have to have a little brown in it to look best. Reds that have a more muted tone, not a clear, vivid tone, are also best for you because you want the red to complement your coloring, not be the main focal point in your make-up. If your hair is medium to dark brown, deep auburn, or salt and pepper and you have brown, hazel or green eyes, you would fall into a category called CPD. A CPD does have a sharp contrast between their hair, eye, and skin color. Therefore, the best red for a CPD would be a red with more depth (not muted because it would look too bright)

and medium intensity. Deeper, brighter reds work best." Giella [Note: See Chapter Four for complete coverage of these color types.]

Red Alert

"My lipstick is so highly pigmented and has that real old-fashioned quality, so I recommend that you put it on right out of the tube. Put the lipstick on first, and then go back later and correct any kind of definition flaw. Each lipstick has a matching pencil; if you don't use a pencil that's complimentary, you can spoil the whole effect of a great red lipstick. Don't put the liner on first or you can end up looking like you have a clown mouth. Use a powder brush on top of the lip line to keep the line crisp and seal it from bleeding. Reverse lining is a trick that makeup artists use. Take a concealer pencil (Julie Hewitt Omit) and use it outside of your lip line. It creates a fleshy highlight against the skin, pops the color on your face, erases errors, and makes your lip line look really crisp." Julie Hewett

Ready for Red?

"If you are afraid to try red lipstick, the best way to start is to line your lips with a nude pencil and then get yourself a sheer red that complements you, or a red gloss, or even a mauve with red in it. Finding the right shade makes it easier to wear red lipstick, and my line has a red for everyone. On the set of *Pearl Harbor*, I used a color similar to Coco Noir, which has brown undertones, and it looked great on everyone. Cooler skintones should stick to blue-reds or true reds, like Rouge Noir or Femme Noir. Rouge Noir is a Technicolor red—the perfect movie-star red that looks great on everyone who loves drama. There's nothing shy about it. Femme Noir is a blue-red that looks beautiful if you have very fair skin with blue undertones. Belle Noir looks amazing on tanned blondes with olive skin, but it also looks good on brunettes with pale olive skin. Sin Noir is a warm eggplanty-red that looks great on Latin women and African Americans—anyone with warmer skintones. I have friends who put it on and wipe it off to wear as a stain because it's so long-lasting. Red lipstick is addictive because it's the one thing that pops your face. That's why our grandmothers wore it. And fortunately, it's really fashionable right now." Julie Hewett

THE PRODUCT FILES

Lip Treatments

The Buzz from the Beauty Editor

I decided to steer clear of balms in this category, since I listed my favorites below, and pick more unusual treatment products, from exfoliants to plumpers. For best results, use a lip exfoliant or mask two to three times a week, preferably at bedtime. Why? Because if lips are too smooth prior to makeup application, lipstick will not adhere. My favorites are Beauticontrol Lip Appeal, $15, and Mary Kay Satin Lips Set, $18.

What the Pros Choose

I discovered a couple of fabulous new lip treatments when I consulted the pros: Naked Kiss Lip Treatment (Dee DeLuca-Mattos) and Skingenious Sexy Kiss Kit (Shan Albert, who claims this product makes lips smoother, fuller, and less prunelike, and even reduces those dreaded wrinkles around the mouth). Other picks include Smith's Rosebud Salve (Hara Glick), Aveda Lip Replenishment (Shauna Raisch), Vaseline Petroleum Jelly (Meredith Green), Smashbox Lip Treatment (Meg Thompson), Lush Lip Treatment (Mala Elhassan), and Aquaphor (Debra Luftman).

Lip Balms (Clear)

The Buzz from the Beauty Editor

I am obsessed with lip balm. I'm never without at least a couple in my bag, and I'm constantly reapplying it whenever I'm at home. I have different lip balms to match my moods: for luxury, it's Acqua di Parma Relaxing Orange Lip Balm, $27, or Fresh Sugar Lip Balm SPF15, $22; for practicality, it's Blistex Clear Advance, $1.99, and Prada Shielding Balm SPF15/Lip, $38; and for intense hydration, I choose Laura Mercier Lip Silk, $20, or Clinique Superbalm Lip Treatment, $11.50. To ease chronically dry lips, make lip balm part of your evening routine. I apply mine right after I brush my teeth. Make sure your lips are dry first, or balm won't go on smoothly and chapped lips will get worse, not better. Also, keep a lip balm in every room in the house so that you can apply it whenever you think of it. (I do the same thing with hand cream.)

What the Pros Choose

Once again, the experts are all over the board. Some picks are surprising, like Lansinoh Nipple Cream (Wende Zomnir) and Elizabeth Arden Eight-Hour Cream (Mala Elhassan), and some more conventional, like Caudalie Lip Conditioner (Julie Hewett) and Smith's Rosebud Salve (Danielle Browning and Hara

Glick). June Jacobs chooses her Lip Silk, while Debra Luftman picks Neostrata AHA with SPF. One beauty insider, Dee DeLuca-Mattos, chooses Chapstick with SPF 15, while another, Gabrielle Ophals, chooses Blistex ProCare. Shauna Raisch selects Aveda Lip Replenishment; Galit Strugano picks The Balm; Meredith Green chooses Kiehl's #1 Lip Balm; and Meg Thompson chooses La Mer The Lip Balm.

Lip Balms (Tinted)

The Buzz from the Beauty Editor

Tinted lip balms let me fool myself into thinking I'm the "fresh-scrubbed, looks-great-in-a-ponytail, low-maintenance type" that I'm definitely not. No low-maintenance girl would have dozens of these, and I do. I love them when I want it to seem as if I'm wearing no makeup at all. For a low-maintenance look that's still polished, try lining your lips and filling them in all over with a neutral lip pencil, like MAC Spice. Your lip balm will have something to adhere to, and your lips will have greater definition. My favorites are Lucky Chick Lucky Lips Lip Shine in a flavor called Mimosa, Jasmine, and Violet, $11, and Bonne Bell Lip Lix in I Scream, $3.50.

What the Pros Choose

Three pros pick Aveda SPF 15 Lip Tint: Julie Hewett, Meg Thompson, and Shauna Raisch, who cites Berry as her favorite color; and two pick Kiehl's: Galit Strugano and Mala Elhassan. Other choices include Lancôme (Dee DeLuca-Mattos), Philosophy Kiss Me (Hara Glick), and Urban Decay Lube in a Tube in New York (Wende Zomnir).

Lipsticks

The Buzz from the Beauty Editor

Lipstick is my favorite makeup product. It's a classic, feminine accessory—and the quickest way to transform a face. Plus, lipstick equals confidence. Try asking for a promotion without it. In lipstick, as in clothing, dark colors reduce while light colors expand. For fuller lips, stick with lighter, shimmery shades, or apply a dab of gloss in the center of your lower lip. My favorite lipsticks are MAC Matte Lipstick in Viva Glam, $14, and Vincent Longo Gel-X Lipstick in Rush, $23.

What the Pros Choose

More of the experts choose MAC as their favorite lipstick than any other brand, including Galit Strugano, June Jacobs, and Meredith Green. Lao cites the color selection as her main reason for putting MAC first. Meg Thompson picks MAC Spirit and Cherish as two of her favorite, universally flattering neutrals, and puts Stila Jane lipstick in that same category, but her absolute favorite shade is NARS Hot Voodoo. Chantecaille is next in line, with Debra Luftman and Julie Hewett rating it tops. Hewett also chooses her own Julie Hewett Noir lipstick, while Debra Macki rates her Heiress shade number one. Lilly Rivera is a big fan of Laura Mercier lipsticks. Her favorite shades are Plum, Baby Lips, and Rosewater. Other choices include Aveda Lip Color Sheer in Sheer Ginseng (Shauna Raisch), NARS Dolce Vita (Hara Glick), and Stila Darla (Dee DeLuca-Mattos).

Liquid Lipsticks

The Buzz from the Beauty Editor

It's sometimes hard to draw the line between a gloss and a liquid lipstick. The best liquid lipsticks combine the color of a lipstick with the shine of a gloss, though there are some notable exceptions. Part of the confusion lies with the industry itself, which may dub an ultra-sheer formulation a "lipstick" and a heavily pigmented formula a "gloss." I try to disregard the cosmetic companies' labels, and choose products with intense, lipstick-like color and, in most cases, shine. It's always a good idea to apply a lipliner before a liquid lipstick. Otherwise, things could get messy. Lining lips and filling them in with a suitable neutral or a matching shade keeps color where it belongs, and helps it last longer. My favorites are Lancôme Lip Dimension Lasting Liquid Lip-Shaping Colour in Rouge Bombe, $20, and New York Color Liquid Lipstick in Christine, $3.99.

What the Pros Choose

Liquid lipsticks can be tricky, even for pros, but that doesn't stop our experts from choosing a few of their favorites, from Bloom Lip Lacquer (Debra Luftman) to Max Factor Lipfinity (Julie Hewett). Shauna Raisch reaches for Aveda Lip Glaze in Mango Juice, and Shan Albert claims that Colorescience Lip Polish imparts the most natural and long-lasting lip color.

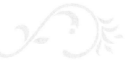

Long-Wearing Lipcolors

The Buzz from the Beauty Editor

Truly long-wearing lipcolors, like Max Factor Lipfinity, Cover Girl Outlast, and Lip Ink Classic Lip Color, all pretty much follow the same formula: you apply a gluey coat of color, wait for it to dry, then finish up with a balm or gloss for moisture and shine. If you can't stand the dehydrating effect of a conventional long-wearing lipstick, or if you prefer a creamier finish, choose a more traditional long-wearing lipstick, such as those from Dior and Chanel, or an ultra-matte lipstick, like Smashbox Limitless Lip Cream. Many long-wearing lipsticks now offer impressive wear. My favorites are Max Factor Lipfinity Everlites in Tickled, $11, and Smashbox Limitless Lip Cream in Infrared, $18.

What the Pros Choose

Most experts decline to pick a long-wearing lipstick, but with new formulas appearing almost daily, this may soon change. A couple of exceptions: both Lilly Rivera and Meg Thompson choose MAC Pro Longwear Lipcolour. Rivera also chooses Lip Sense Lip Color in Rose. Other pros pick lip stains or regular lipsticks that wear well, like Aveda Lip Color Concentrate in Rambutan (Shauna Raisch), NARS (Dee DeLuca-Mattos), and Neutrogena (Debra Luftman).

Lip Stains

The Buzz from the Beauty Editor

For my lip stain choices, I stuck to gel or liquid stains that leave long-lasting, natural, matte pigment on your lips, rather than the glossy sheer lipsticks that are also occasionally dubbed stains. I also stuck to natural red stains—the shade most of us wish came naturally. While some exfoliation may be necessary before applying a lip stain, there is such a thing as lips that are too silky and smooth. If you buff your lips until the surface is sleek and slippery, lipstick and lip stain won't have anything to adhere to. That's why I prefer to exfoliate my lips at bedtime. The next morning, lips won't be too slick, and lipstick and lip stain will go on more evenly. My favorites are Philosophy The Supernatural Lip & Cheek Tint in Super Red, $15, and Sephora Lip Marker in Strawberry, $10.

What the Pros Choose

Experts polled vary widely on stellar stains—ranging from NARS (Dee DeLuca-Mattos) to Delux Beauty (Julie Hewett), Stila Lip Rouge (Meg Thompson) to Clinique lipstick (Debra Luftman). Wende Zomnir stays true to Hard Candy Stain & Shine in Piglet, while Shauna Raisch casts her vote for Aveda Lip Tint SPF 15 in Berry.

Lipliners

The Buzz from the Beauty Editor

I'm a big fan of the new reverse lipliners, which are similar to concealer pencils but designed to be used around the lips. (Julie Hewett's tip at the beginning of the chapter gives guidelines for using these.) I think every woman should have a great neutral liner, for its versatility, and a great red liner, a must for achieving a classic red lip. Line lips after you apply lipstick for a more natural look. This also prevents the lipstick from wearing off first and leaving the liner behind in an unattractive line around your lips. If you are skipping lipstick and using liner alone, apply liner to the inside of the lips first and work out towards the edges. Rest your elbow on something solid for stability, then proceed to line, starting in the center of the upper lip and working out towards the sides using small, feathery strokes. If your natural lip line is undefined, as mine is, err by lining a little on the inside rather than the outside. You can always take the line out farther, but wiping off an overdrawn lipline is trickier. Also, lining lips a little narrow rather than a little full avoids the floppy, clownlike, too-much-collagen look too many women are sporting. My favorite liners are Lancôme Le Lipstique in Rougelle, $20, and Julie Hewett Omit Pencil, $12.

What the Pros Choose

Once again, this category is proof that, even among experts, consensus is hard to come by. MAC gets the most votes: June Jacobs, Meredith Green, Meg Thompson (Spice), and Lilly Rivera (Spice, Plum, Chestnut, and Cork). Other favorites include Paula Dorf Antique (Hara Glick), Aveda Lip Liner in Kantola Bean (Shauna Raisch), Pout in 34C (Galit Strugano), NARS Morocco (Dee DeLuca-Mattos), and Prescriptives (Debra Luftman). Shan Albert loves Colorescience's Life's a Peach and Tickled Pink. Naturally, a couple of the pros like their own formulas best: Julie Hewett picks her Nude Noir, and Debra Macki picks her Sand liner.

Lip Glosses

The Buzz from the Beauty Editor

Lip gloss can range from sheer and natural to dramatic and color-drenched. For darker or brighter colors, I generally stick to a lipstick, as it's less messy, easier to apply, and longer-lasting. I prefer my gloss in a sheer pink or nude shade with some subtle shimmer—never glitter—for a look that's full and fabulous. I also like the sheer reds and berries that are sometimes referred to as stains. If they're sheer, shiny, and have limited staying power, they're a gloss, in my opinion, no matter what the label says. Whatever you call them, they're a quick choice for a shot of color without a lot of fuss. Don't apply gloss (or lipstick, for that matter) too close to the inside of your lip, where your lips touch your teeth. You'll get gloss all over your teeth, and after a few hours, you'll have that unappealing, gummy white line around the inside perimeter of your lips. My favorite glosses are Sebastian Trucco Divinyls in Baby Doll, $11, Clinique Glosswear in Tender Heart, $13.50, and Bloom Lipgloss in Tint, $17.

What the Pros Choose

Two experts rank MAC first: Hara Glick loves the classic clear Lipglass, and Lilly Rivera loves all the shades. Rivera also chooses her own BridalGal Boutique glosses in Clear and Baby Doll, BridalGal Boutique Line 'n Lacquer gloss and liner duo in Crystal Pink/Charmed, and Laura Mercier glosses in Violet Glaze, Rose, and Bare Beige. Rivera isn't the only expert to choose a gloss called Baby Doll: different formulas bearing the same-named shade are chosen by Dee DeLuca-Mattos (Sebastian Trucco Divinyls) and

Meg Thompson (NARS Lip Lacquer). Thompson loves NARS Lip Lacquers for their creamy finish and color options, and also favors any of Trish McEvoy's glosses for their texture and colors. Chantecaille is the pick of Debra Luftman and Julie Hewett, while Stila is tops with June Jacobs. Danielle Browning has high praise for her pick, Paul & Joe Lip Gloss. It "makes lips look like glass and is not too sticky!" She also loves Cargo's glosses. Fiona Locke also raves about her top choice, California Tan Sunless Lip Shine, "It has plumpers for sexy full lips and a rosy, slightly shimmery tint." More eclectic picks include Urban Decay XXX Shine in Carney (Wende Zomnir), Aveda Lip Shine in Grapefruit Pulp (Shauna Raisch), Debra Macki Lipgloss in Casino (Debra Macki), Girlactik Star Gloss in Super Star Silver (Galit Strugano), Revlon Lipglide in Sheerly Blossom (Meredith Green), Chanel Glossimer (Mala Elhassan), and Love Nectar Potions Honey Rose Kissing Balm (Linda Deslauriers).

Lip Palettes

The Buzz from the Beauty Editor

I love lip palettes for a variety of reasons: they give you a chance to try out colors you might not otherwise use, and they're a portable way to take along a selection of shades. Plus, I love the packaging. I always keep one of the tinier lip palettes (like Trish McEvoy's) and a retractable lip brush in the zippered compartment of my handbag, so that I'm never without the perfect lip shade. My favorite palettes are Smashbox Lip Brilliance in Skybox, $26, and Black Opal Lipcolor Kit in Glazed Berries, $5.25.

What the Pros Choose

The problem with palettes is that companies are continually coming out with new ones and discontinuing old favorites. Still, readers and experts alike hold on to their favorites, even if they are no longer available. Galit Strugano and Meredith Green both choose Stila, with Strugano specifying their limited-edition holiday palettes. Dee DeLuca-Mattos and Hara Glick choose NARS, with Glick singling out the popular Hot Sauce palette. Other picks include Trish McEvoy (Meg Thompson), Aveda Lip Sheers (Shauna Raisch), Tina Earnshaw (Julie Hewett), and Hard Candy Lip Sync in Drama Queen (Wende Zomnir).

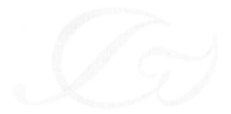

Chapter Seven

Beautiful Body Care:
Pamper Yourself with Self-Indulgent Spa Secrets and Serious Solutions

This is the only category of products designed almost exclusively for pleasure. They have the power to transform a humble bathroom into a luxurious spa. Soap is soap, and one could argue that it's the only really essential body product. But those of us who've fallen under the spell of lotions and creams, washes and scrubs, know better. We know that while any body wash can clean, it takes an exceptional product to soothe our skin and seduce our senses. Picking a body product is a purely personal—completely idiosyncratic—decision, based on how the product feels and how it makes us feel, how it smells and how that smell affects our mood.

THE *Beauty Bunch* BREAKDOWN

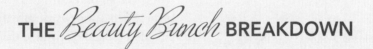

Gabrielle Ophals: cofounder and co-owner of Haven Spa, a serene spot in New York City's hip SoHo neighborhood.

Kathryn Alice: beauty publicist with her own firm, The Alice Company.

June Jacobs: skin-care expert, beauty entrepreneur, and founder of June Jacobs Spa Collection.

Wende Zomnir: creative director of Hard Candy Cosmetics and founder/creative director of Urban Decay Cosmetics.

Meredith Green: publicist and lifestyle expert.

Bettijo B. Hirschi: creator of Bath By Bettijo, a line of natural, handmade bath and body products that have been featured in the pages of *O*, *Allure*, and *Lucky*.

Jeffrey Dover, MD: top dermatologist, professor, and creator of Skin Effects, the first dermatologist-developed anti-aging line for the mass market.

Dee DeLuca-Mattos: vice president of Avancé Skincare.

Angela Nice: skin-care specialist, creator and cofounder of Los Angeles's M Aesthetics Spa, and one of the country's foremost experts in body sculpting and cellulite reduction.

Jessica Wu, MD: Harvard-educated dermatologist and well-known media personality.

BASIC BODY CARE

The Buzz from the Beauty Editor

I am absolutely obsessed with body treatments, and I have been as long as I can remember. In college, my friends teased me because I regularly slathered myself with spa mud and tiptoed around the sorority house in the middle of the night. I can still be found on any given weeknight, covered in a body mask of some kind. Sure, they smooth, silken, and detoxify, but the greatest benefit is in the sheer luxury of pampering yourself.

Insider Information from the Beauty Bunch

Fresh-Scrubbed

"You should exfoliate regularly but not too frequently; one to three times a week is good. Exfoliating is important because you want to make sure that your skin adequately absorbs the nutrients and the beneficial properties of your moisturizer, so you have to make sure that the dead skin cells are removed." Gabrielle Ophals

Warding off Wings

"Getting droopy upper arms? To avoid the 'wings' that older women often get, back up to a chair and grip it with your hands. Lower your body up and down a few times, letting the back of the chair hold your weight. This works the muscles that will keep your upper-arm skin from sagging. Do ten reps twice a day." Kathryn Alice

Scrub and Screen

"Using sunscreen and exfoliating are two of the most important things you can do for your body." June Jacobs

Lasting Luster

"Set body shimmer or glitter with a light misting of aerosol hair spray, especially if you are going dancing. My husband demanded that I figure out a way to keep his tux from getting sparkly, and this works!" Wende Zomnir

Stellar Standby

"Don't leave home without Vaseline Petroleum Jelly. You can use it on your lips, on your cuticles, on your feet—the possibilities are endless!" Meredith Green

Body Brushing

"Exfoliation is a critical step in body care; it boosts skin's natural rejuvenation by sloughing away dry dead skin. Besides leaving your skin soft and glowing, it is also a natural way to rev up your lymphatic system—the body's waste-disposal system—improving its ability to remove built-up toxins. Skin brushing with a dry sisal brush is an age-old, Asian-inspired treatment that is easy to do for yourself. When done regularly, dry brushing can improve your skin's surface circulation and keep pores open, providing healthier and more resilient skin. Benefits range from reduced cellulite to an increased skintone and strengthened immune system. You can find a sisal brush for about fifteen dollars at most quality bath and body boutiques in your neighborhood or online. Brushing should be done on dry skin once a day; it's easy to do right before entering a shower. Always try to brush towards your heart. Brush the soles of your feet first, because the nerve endings there affect the entire body. Next, using an upward motion, brush the ankles, calves, and thighs. Move up to your stomach and buttocks and finish by brushing your hands and arms. Wash your brush every few weeks and let it dry thoroughly before using." Bettijo B. Hirschi

Divine Décolleté

"Use facial products on décolleté. It gets a lot more sun than the rest of your body, and it's a lot more visible, so treat it with the best products." Gabrielle Ophals

SOOTHING SCARS AND STRETCH MARKS

The Buzz from the Beauty Editor

Following a growth spurt as a teen, I found myself with stretch marks on my upper outer thighs. Naturally, I've always hated them, and spent years keeping them under wraps. Today, I conceal them with a little body make-up. Until there's a cure, there's always a way to cover up. For fresh stretch marks, there's still hope. Retin-A, if applied daily for a few months, can help to diminish red stretch marks. Pulsed dye lasers also diminish redness. For older, white stretch marks, infrared lasers can help smooth and refine texture. Unfortunately, while lasers can help, they can't erase the ravages of stretch marks; a 10-percent improvement is considered good.

Insider Information from the Beauty Bunch

Pregnancy Pointer

"If you're pregnant, avoid stretch marks by rubbing the belly with a daily sugar scrub, then massaging in a rich oil—I used Weleda Rose Oil in the morning, then an almond oil blended with lavender and rose-geranium essential oils in the evening." Wende Zomnir

Bumps and Bruises

"There is no effective treatment for bruising except the tincture of time. The best treatment for scars is pulsed dye lasers, although intense pulsed light may work as well. A series of treatments done every four to six weeks is necessary. The more treatments performed, the better the results." Jeffrey Dover, MD

Treating Scars and Stretch Marks

"For fresh, bumpy red scars, you can laser them to get the redness out or inject them with cortisol to flatten them or use a fading cream to get rid of darkness. For old, white scars, there's not much we can do for them. The same is true with stretch marks. If they're new and fresh, they can be treated, but there is not much yet that can be done to treat them if they're older." Jessica Wu, MD

DEFEATING DRYNESS

The Buzz from the Beauty Editor
I never had a problem with dry skin on my body until I lived in Chicago for a couple of years. Suddenly, every winter, my legs would get chronically dry and itchy, and I found myself scratching them until they were red. Finally, I started addressing the problem, cutting down on hot baths and applying rich creams and oils morning and night. And I stopped scratching. Soon, I had the dryness under control.

Insider Information from the Beauty Bunch

Essential Moisture
"Most of us are totally dehydrated. Stop drinking Diet Coke and drink water. It can make a difference in your skin's moisture level and cellulite appearance, and improves skin's overall quality." Gabrielle Ophals

Dry Skin Eliminator
"If you have really dry skin, slather baby oil or even Vaseline [Petroleum Jelly] on after you shower and before you towel off. They are the only things I've found that work to keep my superdry skin moist.

I've never had any adverse effects, and my skin glows." Kathryn Alice

Damp, Not Dry
"When showering, especially in the winter, do not completely dry your skin. Pat dry with a towel, and use Avancé Toning Body Crème when your body is damp. This assists in not only maintaining the moisture in the skin, but it also adds maximum moisture to the entire body." Dee DeLuca-Mattos

Skin Softening
"I have a friend who is psychotic about moisturizing. We've gone on vacation together and it's annoying because she is in the bathroom forever, but her skin is baby soft. She gets out of the shower and moisturizes from head to toe; it goes on every spot her hands can reach. If your skin is healthy and nourished, it will enhance and lengthen its life, and you'll be less prone to stretch marks. Use a quality moisturizer and apply it right out of the shower. Even the mineral-oil lotions are better than nothing. At least they are providing a barrier for your skin." Gabrielle Ophals

Chronic Dryness
"Make sure there's nothing you're doing to cause dry skin, like using strong deodorant or antibacterial soaps, and that you're not taking too many showers, like two to three a day. Don't do anything to make it worse. Some people have very dry skin in the winter or in drier climates. Olay has a great new product called Moisturinse In Shower Body Lotion. It's got petrolatum in it, and it's like conditioner for your skin. After you get out of the shower, make sure to seal in the moisture. Pat dry and apply moisturizer. I also recommend Neutrogena Sesame Body Oil. If you have areas of flakiness, exfoliate with a lotion like LacHydrin, which is a prescription lotion with glycolic acid." Jessica Wu, MD

Feed Your Body

"Use moisturizers with nourishing oils. Look at the ingredient list. Make sure that you don't see mineral oil in the first three ingredients. It's not the devil, but it's just not that nourishing. Inexpensive body lotions will use mineral oil because it's cheap. You want to heal dry skin, not just cover up the problem with greasiness. Look for a phytobotanical oil, an oil that is derived from plants, in the first few ingredients. Shea butter is a great nourishing, hydrating ingredient. Check to see that it is in the first three or four ingredients. Jojoba oil is another nourishing ingredient; it is chemically very similar to our own natural oils, so that our skin recognizes it and absorbs it easily. Oils that are derived from fruit, like coconut, avocado, or peach oils, are also very nourishing. A good body lotion with quality ingredients tends to be a little more expensive, but you are getting a product that is better for your skin. Your skin is a living organism and you need to feed it." Gabrielle Ophals

Moisturizer Matters

"Moisturizers are effective on all parts of the body. The only difference is a person's personal choice. Most prefer a slightly lighter product for the arms and body and a slightly thicker cream for the neck and face. The best treatment for chronically dry skin is moisturization. This is best applied in the bath using a non-suspension product. Some of my favorites include Aveeno oilated bath or oatmeal flakes, and Keri Oil. Topicals which are effective include twelve-percent—but not five-percent—lactic acid [and] are available both over-the-counter and by prescription. There are also a variety of other topical agents which include ceramides, which are lipid-laden spherules within the cream or lotion which help to hydrate the skin. This needs to be done once or preferably twice a day immediately after bathing, or [after] a shower when the skin is still damp and when penetration is best. Products work as humectants by drawing water from the dermis into the upper dermis, naturally helping to rehydrate the skin." Jeffrey Dover, MD

Scent Selection

"First, pick a scent that you like. Then, make sure that your body lotion contains essential oils and not fragrance oils. Otherwise, you are not getting the beneficial properties, and it will not affect your mood the way you expect it to. It may smell like lavender, but if the body lotion is two to three dollars for eight ounces and the ingredient list contains fragrance oils, it will not have the beneficial effects you associate with lavender, such as relaxing and relieving stress. That's why you commonly find fragrance oils in inexpensive body lotions; they are much cheaper than essential oils. Essential oils are actually chemicals that are extracted from the plants. You won't get the benefits of the plant if you don't actually use the plant." Gabrielle Ophals

CELLULITE STRATEGIES

The Buzz from the Beauty Editor

Even though my body can best be described as scrawny, I still suffer from cellulite on the backs of my thighs. Apparently, I'm in good company, because 90 percent of women have the same problem. It takes a commitment of time and money to tackle cellulite, but fortunately, treatments exist that can drastically improve your bottom line. Read on for details.

Insider Information from the Beauty Bunch

Cellulite Science

"I am very wary of cellulite products; I just don't see how slathering on a body lotion is going to get rid of fat. Many of them contain menthol or camphor and they can be cooling and produce a tightening effect, but any benefits are rinsed off in the shower. Many cellulite products come with massagers, and self-massage is very healthy because it can help break fat down, but it's the massage, not the product, that's beneficial." Gabrielle Ophals

Cellulite Solutions

"Regular massages or deep-tissue massage is what makes a cellulite cream work effectively. Look for ingredients like niacin or a caffeine derivative when shopping for a cellulite cream. I am currently using a new one with six years of research behind it called Cellulite Rx. It's a three-step process, with a body polish, a contour cream, and a firming cream. The contour cream has some progesterone, niacin, and caffeine, for blood circulation and stimulation. It increases circulation like nothing I've never seen before. Skin is warm and red and tingly for about an hour after application. It's a very, very advanced product. You need to wash your hands afterwards, or they get sensitive and red. You don't need to use much, and you need to really massage it in until you feel it's fully absorbed. It is a vasodilator, so it really increases the circulation of the body to flush out toxins from your cells. The third cream is a collagen stimulator. It feels and smells peppery. Some people use it before and after Endermologie, an FDA-approved, professionally administered treatment which uses a motorized device to target cellulite. The trademark ingredient is a QuSome liposome-delivery system. I've had wonderful results using this in conjunction with Endermologie. It wasn't enough by itself." Angela Nice

Weighty Solutions

"Weight-bearing exercise is the most important thing you can do to conquer cellulite. A lot of women who lose a lot of weight also lose a lot of muscle. Skin doesn't look as healthy and elastic as it used to. Weight-bearing exercise is the number-one thing they need to do. Muscle replaces fat cells. Resistance training, like Pilates or yoga, helps too, because you engage the muscles. Muscle-building is what blows up fat cells and cellulite cells." Angela Nice

Top Treatment

"I like Endermologie. It's the gold standard, without a doubt. Plus it feels good and therapeutic. It has FDA approval for the appearance of cellulite, and it helps blood flow to be even throughout the body. It is the most effective at breaking apart adhesions and fibroblasts that attach themselves to fat cells. It is the best modality to break apart these colonies that are underneath the skin. We have also been using Delasmooth, which is sort of like Endermologie with radio frequency and infrared. It penetrates deeper, and it helps to melt the fat so the body can reabsorb it better. I like it better than Triactive [an alternate cellulite treatment]. The results [of Triactive] are nice, but most people preferred Endermologie. All require a series of treatments. Endermologie requires fourteen to twenty sessions, while the Delasmooth [another cellulite treatment] needs ten to fourteen sessions. It is normal to have some bruising, and it can be painful, but it's tolerable. If you want it to be perfect, you need to keep having the treatments. If I also use a cellulite cream, I can go about three weeks. But ideally, I like to go every week to look my best. They help to balance the hormones and they also keep the circulation going and get rid of water weight. Other treatments that are supposed to address cellulite are Ionothermie and body wraps, but they don't really work. You lose inches right away, but you gain them back right away, too." Angela Nice

Home Care

"There is a new product called the Wellbox. It's an at-home treatment similar to Endermologie, and it's made by the same company. It's patented; some companies knock it off, but they don't work as well. [With the knockoffs] skin can get twisted or pinched or bruised. They're worse than the Epilady. There have been problems in the past with at-home cellulite techniques, but the Wellbox is different. It's promising." Angela Nice

Water Works

"Massage is always nice, and drinking a lot of water is key. Drink two quarts of water a day. A lot of women lose somewhere between five to eight pounds their first and second weeks just by drinking water and using Endermologie. You will go to the bathroom a lot, and lose toxins. After about ten days, it normalizes, and your body starts using it for organs. It makes all the difference in the world for general health. If you have a problem drinking enough water, try lemon or cucumber water. Lemon and cucumber are purifiers and diuretics. One slice of cucumber will flavor a giant pitcher of water, and you can keep adding water to it all day long. We have salad water here every day. You can put anything in it: strawberries, cherries, green beans, rosemary, mint. Drink out of a straw. Buy different sizes or different kinds of water. Any of these things can help." Angela Nice

Lunge Lowdown

"Diet is important, but it's not as important as exercise. Number one is the lunge. Number two is the squat. At the gym, you can do a series of exercises that we call the fives. You do the in and out machines for inner and outer thighs; the leg press for the whole area, which just blows the cellulite right out of the skin; the leg lift for your quads; and the curl, where you curl it back into the hamstring. Then you're covered. It doesn't take much weight, but it has to be weight bearing. And try taking the stairs. These are all choices that you can make throughout the day that can make a big difference in the shape of your body." Angela Nice

Slimming Sneakers

"I like the Swiss Masai sneakers from MBT. I'm wearing them now as I speak. They're based on the Masai tribe in Africa which has always walked on an uneven surface. They take a little balance. You have to constantly use your core muscles; it's a constant workout. You should ease into wearing them. I love them. I find them very comfortable, and you can definitely see a difference." Angela Nice

SPA SPEAK

The Buzz from the Beauty Editor

Spas are my natural habitat. I am most at home in them, and there isn't a single spa treatment that I haven't tried. A few years ago, the day before my wedding, I treated myself, my eight bridesmaids, and my mother to a spa day at the Breakers in Palm Beach. Between treatments, we lounged around in our robes on the spa's private patio and nibbled on spa lunches. For the spa veterans and novices alike, it was a luxurious, pampering way to kick off the wedding weekend—and it was one of the best days of my life.

Insider Information from the Beauty Bunch

Spa Assessment

"I think it depends on what you are going in there for. Sit down and talk and consult and [let them] see what you are trying to achieve. Also, how do you feel when you leave? When you go home and look at your skin, you should see the results. Voice your opinion, speak up, and let them know what could work or might not." Wende Zomnir

Body Treatments for Beginners

"In a nutshell, body treatments involve getting naked on a bed and getting scrubbed or rubbed. You get on the table, there's a scrubbing action, and then what I call the marination phase, which involves a clay or seaweed or herbal wrap. Then you are rinsed and moisturized. Today, many of them are based on food, like chocolate or coconut or fruit. Look at the menu and pick something that looks fun to you. Don't be shy or embarrassed to ask questions. Most of the time, they expect that it is your first time and that you don't know what is happening. Call and ask questions before you make an appointment; if they are reluctant or unable to answer questions, that's a red flag. They should be willing and able, and if the person on the phone doesn't have the answers, they should make sure that they find someone who can answer your questions. If they don't, that's scary; you want to feel comfortable." Gabrielle Ophals

Salt or Sugar

"Salt glows are the most basic body treatments. Personally, I am not a huge fan of them because I feel they can be a little abrasive, but many people love them. Salt and sugar scrubs are essentially the same thing; they are just different carriers. The only real difference is that salt is detoxifying, so you can't use it on a pregnant woman." Gabrielle Ophals

Home Spa

"A body scrub is one of the most popular spa treatments with almost instant results. It leaves you with baby-soft skin, but also provides lasting benefits by stimulating circulation and skin-cell renewal. While it is definitely a real treat to have a body polish done for you, it is simple and rewarding to do at home. Try this basic body scrub recipe at home. Combine half a cup of salt or sugar—use sugar if your skin is more sensitive—half a cup of olive oil, and thirty drops essential oil of sweet orange or peppermint. Both have invigorating and energizing properties, but you can also sub your favorite. Put the ingredients in a plastic bowl for safety, in case it slips out of your hands in the shower. Begin your shower by wetting your skin from head to toe, then step out of the water stream to apply your body polish. Using an upward motion, scrubbing towards your heart, buff your feet, legs, thighs, and stomach and finish with your arms and hands. Do not use this scrub on delicate facial skin. Step carefully back under the water flow—the skin-nourishing oils might make the shower floor a bit slippery—and rinse completely. Now bask in your exquisitely smooth and beautiful skin!" Bettijo B. Hirschi

Modest Maneuvers

"Body treatments are different from massages in that there are typically not that many modesty considerations, because they originated in Europe where modesty standards are different. We don't advise bathing suits during body treatments; we provide disposable panties, and if it makes you more comfortable, a towel across the breasts. Some clients don't want the towel. Our therapists are advised to ask whether or not you want the exfoliation on your breasts. When you make the appointment, ask about a male or female therapist. Request the one that makes you comfortable." Gabrielle Ophals

Questions and Comments

"Ask as many questions as you want to during a body treatment or massage. You can also ask for a silent treatment if you don't want the treatment explained to you or don't feel like chatting. One of the biggest challenges in the industry is people feeling shy and not wanting to hurt feelings. If you don't like a lot of pressure, don't ask for a deep-tissue massage. Specify if it's your first massage." Gabrielle Ophals

THE PRODUCT FILES

Body Washes

The Buzz from the Beauty Editor

When my friend Carla visited from Holland several years ago, she was astonished to find soap in my bathroom. In Europe, soap had long been shunned in favor of skin-friendly shower gels, but in the United States, shower gels were just catching on. (Shower gels only became popular in the U.S. after they were sold with scrubbing aids. Apparently, Americans don't like to touch their own bodies.) However, once I started using shower gels, I never looked back. They are gentler, less drying, and more luxurious than soaps. I still buy soap, but now I only buy beautifully packaged scented soaps to adorn a bathroom or to slip into drawers to add fragrance. When traveling, I often use a moisturizing shower gel, like Clinique Skin Cushion, in place of a shaving cream. One less bottle to pack. My favorites are Mario Russo Olive Juice, $18, and Olay Moisturinse In Shower Body Lotion, $7.

What the Pros Choose

Sudsing up in the shower is something the pros take seriously, and each has specific ideas about the best product for the job. Two pros opt for products that are free of sodium laurel sulfate, Wende Zomnir's The Organic Sudz Company Tour de Body Wash in Honey Pot and Shan Albert's Franché CranMary Purifying Body Foam. Other picks include Aveda Energizing Body Cleanser (Shauna Raisch), Bath & Body Works (Meredith Green), Fresh Milk Shower Foam (Mala Elhassan), California North Gelskin Wash (Jim Miller), Peter Thomas Roth Glycolic Acid 3% Shower and Body Cleansing Gel (Peter Thomas Roth), June Jacobs Grapefruit Shower Gel (June Jacobs), Avancé Hydrating Body Wash (Dee DeLuca-Mattos), and The Vital Image Face and Body Wash (Linda Deslauriers). Meg Thompson has perhaps the most surprising pick: Baby Magic Baby Wash.

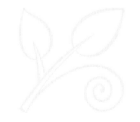

Scrubs and Exfoliators

The Buzz from the Beauty Editor

I have a love-hate relationship with body scrubs. I love the almost edible scents and the pleasurable pampering of using a scrub, but I hate the greasy residue in my tub and the effort they sometimes take to apply. When I do reach for a scrub, I want it to work miracles. I choose sugar scrubs over salt scrubs because they are gentler and less irritating, and sugar is said to combat body breakouts. As an alternative to body scrubs, try mitts and loofahs that turn your everyday shower gel into an exfoliating treatment. My top picks are the gloves that sell everywhere for around five dollars (Earth Therapeutics calls them Exfoliating Hydro Gloves) that fit snugly over both hands to cleanse and exfoliate at the same time. Anywhere your fingers can reach, these gloves can exfoliate, and they won't slip away in the shower. Also, they last practically forever, making them way more budget-friendly than high-priced scrubs. Whether you choose mitts or scrubs, remember that overexfoliation leads to irritation. No matter how yummy, limit the use of strong scrubs to a couple of times a week. My favorite scrubs are The Organic Bath Company Daily Body Scrub White Tea No. 22, $7.50, and Fresh Brown Sugar Body Polish, $62.50. I also love some of the more innovative new exfoliators out there, like DermaNew Crystal Resurfacing Soap, $20, and MD Skincare Alpha Beta Daily Body Peel, $78.

What the Pros Choose

Dessert seems to be on everyone's minds for this category. Sweet scrubs include Tahitian Coconut Milk Scrub (Julie Hewett), Peter Thomas Roth Strawberry Scrub (Peter Thomas Roth), June Jacobs Mandarin Polishing Beads (June Jacobs), Issimo Relax! Niaouli & Carrot Merengue (Meredith Green), and Urban Decay Joe Glow Head-to-Toe Caffeinated Scrub and Wash (Wende Zomnir). Other choices include California Tan Sunless Primer (Fiona Locke's pick because it doesn't contain oils that can interfere with a sunless tan), Enessa Body Polish (Michelle Ornstein), Aveda Smoothing Body Polish (Shauna Raisch), Haven Bamboo Scrub (Gabrielle Ophals), Peter Thomas Roth Botanical Buffing Beads (another choice from June Jacobs), Avancé Hydrating Body Polish (Dee DeLuca-Mattos), Blisslabs Hot Salt Scrub (Charles Worthington), California North Gelskin Scrub (Jim Miller), Origins (Meg Thompson), and SkinCeuticals Body Polish (Debra Luftman).

Bubble Baths

The Buzz from the Beauty Editor

I adore long, leisurely soaks in the tub. Nothing is more relaxing, more therapeutic, or more feminine. When I don't have a bath for a few days, my mood is noticeably worse, so much so that, when renovating the "hers" bathroom in our master suite recently, my husband insisted on having the tub installed and fully functional long before the rest of the room was done. For months, I stepped over broken tiles and cleared away power tools as I made my way to my brand-new bathtub for a much-needed soak, and it was well worth it. Hot baths may be enjoyable, but they can be hard on your skin. Also, they can leave you feeling drained rather than refreshed. Ideally, a bath should be moderately hot, not scalding, and brief—about fifteen minutes. Too much longer and skin is dry and irritable. My favorites are Dirty Girl Bubble Bath, $11.95, and Caswell-Massey New York Bath Tub Gin, $26.

lotion almost immediately after your shower. Dab off the excess moisture on your body (don't rub vigorously) and apply lotion liberally to arms, legs, and other flake-prone areas to prevent dryness. My favorites are Palmer's Skin Success Eventone Fade Milk, $8.60, and La Mer The Body Serum, $150.

What the Pros Choose

Picks in this category range from the therapeutic, like California North Appellation Spa Therapeutic Grapeseed Muscle Soak (Jim Miller), The Thymes Limited SleepWell Epsom Bath Salts (Meg Thompson), and Avancé Stress Relief Sea Bath (Dee DeLuca-Mattos), to the simply indulgent, like Aveda Caribbean Therapy Bath Soak (Shauna Raisch), and both of Wende Zomnir's picks, California Baby Calming Bubble Bath and Laura Mercier Honey Bath. But by far the most unusual pick comes from Kathryn Alice: a Neti Pot picked up in Chinatown. "Every day, the Chinese bathe their sinuses while in the shower or bath using this contraption. You use water with a little sea salt dissolved in it. It hurts if you have sinus infections, but it clears any sinus problems up and does away with the dark circles under the eye that result from sinus problems."

Body Lotions

The Buzz from the Beauty Editor

I have high expectations for my body lotions. They either have to smell and feel amazingly indulgent and luxurious, or they have to be real workhorses—smoothing, refining, and clarifying skin. Some even do both. Your skin loses its moisture within three minutes of taking a bath or shower, so it's best to apply your body

What the Pros Choose

There are hundreds of body lotions out there, so I guess it's no surprise that there is no repetition in this category. The winning lotions could be divided into a few categories, however. "Natural" lotions, with naturally inspired and derived formulas and some fruit or plant ingredients, include Biotone Pomegranate & Cranberry Hydrating Lotion (Gabrielle Ophals), Weleda Aloe Vera Lotion (Wende Zomnir), June Jacobs Spa Collection Citrus Body Balm (June Jacobs), Franché CranMary Hand and Body Smoothie Lotion (Shan Albert), and Kiehl's Coriander Lotion (Meredith Green). "Treatment" lotions, which focus on skin-saving ingredients like AHAs and antioxidants, include California North Action Moisturizer (Jim Miller), which is oil-free and packed with grapeseed extract; and Peter Thomas Roth AHA 12% Body Lotion (Peter Thomas Roth). "Luxury" lotions include Santa Maria Novella Body Milk (Meg Thompson); La Mer (Julie Hewett); and Jo Malone Lime, Basil & Mandarin (Charles Worthington). Other picks are Aveda Replenishing Body Moisturizer (Shauna Raisch), Fresh Milk Body Lotion (Mala Elhassan), Henri Bendel (Danielle Browning), Victoria's Secret (Galit Strugano), Avancé Hydrating Body Lotion (Dee DeLuca-Mattos), and Aveeno Moisturizing Lotion (Debra Luftman).

Body Creams

What the Pros Choose

A lot of fruity creams turn up on this list: June Jacobs Citrus Body Balm (June Jacobs), Trish McEvoy Super Rich Body Balm in Blackberry Vanilla (Danielle Browning), Blisslabs Lemon & Sage Body Butter (Charles Worthington), and Issimo Relax! Valerian and Sweet Orange Crème (Meredith Green). Shan Albert loves Franché CranMary Ultimate Cream. "It's rich, luscious and smells incredibly good. It contains cranberry to protect the skin and rosemary to revitalize. The ingredients are fabulous: milk extracts, shea butter, olive oil, vitamins A and E, Beta fructan—which helps the skin moisturize itself. I love it because it leaves the skin feeling incredibly soft with no greasy feel." Wende Zomnir's pick is Osmotics Tri-Ceram; Julie Hewett craves La Mer; Shauna Raisch likes Aveda Caribbean Therapy Body Crème; and Dee DeLuca-Mattos chooses Avancé Toning Body Crème. Michelle Ornstein prefers an oil, specifically Enessa After Bath Body Oil.

Intensive Moisturizers

What the Pros Choose

Wende Zomnir makes Weleda Wild Rose Oil her choice, while Michelle Ornstein selects Enessa Palm Cream. For extra moisture, Debra Luftman turns to RoC Enydrial Moisturizing Cream, and Shauna Raisch reaches for Aveda Intense Hydrating Masque.

Chapter Eight

Safe Sun Solutions:
Safeguard Your Skin with the Inside Scoop on Sun Protection

This chapter is the one of the shortest, but don't let that fool you. If you read nothing else in this book, you need to read this. Sun protection is one of the few areas where beauty and health meet, and where what you don't know can hurt you. Sunscreen is the single most important step in your skin-care routine, and the only step guaranteed to ward off a slew of skin disorders, from wrinkles to hyperpigmentation, dryness to roughness. It's also the only thing that can ward off more sinister skin woes, like skin cancer. This chapter covers only two categories: sunscreens, for that critical sun protection; and self-tanners, for those who want to have it made in the shade.

THE *Beauty Bunch* BREAKDOWN

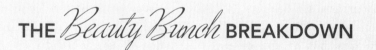

Rebecca James Gadberry: the professional skin-care industry's leading ingredient expert.

Peter Thomas Roth: skin-care entrepreneur with an eponymous skin-care line.

June Jacobs: skin-care expert, beauty entrepreneur, and founder of June Jacobs Spa Collection.

Dennis Gross, MD: Manhattan-based dermatologist, creator of MD Skincare, and author of *Your Future Face*.

Jan Marini: skin-care authority and founder of Jan Marini Skin Research.

Jim Miller: founder of California North, a West Coast skin-care line.

Giella: professional makeup artist and founder of GIELLA Custom Blend Cosmetics.

Mary Lupo, MD: one of the country's foremost dermatologists, she is also a professor at Tulane University Medical School, a frequent television personality, and a skin-care entrepreneur.

Jeffrey Dover, MD: top dermatologist, professor, and creator of Skin Effects, the first dermatologist-developed anti-aging line for the mass market.

Rick Noodleman, MD: cosmetic dermatologist, cocreator of Revercel anti-aging skin-care products, and medical director of Age Defying Dermatology, the largest cosmetic surgery medical center in Silicon Valley.

Jessica Wu, MD: Harvard-educated dermatologist and well-known media personality.

Kathryn Alice: beauty publicist with her own firm, The Alice Company.

Clarissa Azar: one of the founders of Fake Bake, a premier line of self-tanning products favored by Britney Spears and Madonna.

Fiona Locke: senior spray technician, California Tan Sunless Spray Tanning System.

Angela Nice: skin-care specialist, creator and cofounder of Los Angeles's M Aesthetics Spa, and one of the country's foremost experts in body sculpting and cellulite reduction.

SUNSCREEN SAVVY

The Buzz from the Beauty Editor

Even though I have olive skin that tans and never burns, I've been obsessed with sun protection since college. Fortunately, my vanity has paid off, and I have minimal sun damage. I live in Florida, so I never leave my bathroom in the morning without a generous coating of sunscreen on my body and my face. Even though I work at home, I know that UVA rays can find me through the windows. On indoor days, I use a light sunscreen on my face. On errand-running days, I up the SPF. I never sit or lay out in the sun, preferring to swim in the evening and take cover under floppy hats and sunglasses. And I make sure to use enough sunscreen: a full shot glass—or an ounce—of sunscreen to cover my body, and a teaspoon for my face.

Insider Information from the Beauty Bunch

Translating Sunscreens

"I like zinc oxide the best because it's multifunctional and soothing. It's on the skin protectant and the anti-acne monographs. If it's not micronized too finely, it has a very broad spectrum that can protect the skin from ultraviolet lights all the way to the invisible light spectrum. I also like titanium dioxide. It doesn't have as broad a spectrum as zinc oxide, but it works well on UVB rays and lower-level UVA rays. I'm not a fan of UVA-absorbing sunscreens, like avobenzone (Parsol 1789), octyl methoxycinnamate (Parsol MCX), and benzophenone because I find them to be irritants." Rebecca James Gadberry

Waiting Period

"Some people say that they tan through an SPF 30; that usually means you are not putting enough on. You need full coverage. Don't apply it like you are using moisturizer. And you have to wait thirty minutes before going out, or for the first thirty minutes you are unprotected, unless your sunblock contains titanium dioxide. Unlike chemical sunscreens, titanium-dioxide sunscreen protects immediately. You can put it on and go right out. After you apply sunscreen, wait a few minutes for it to absorb and then rub it in again and most of the sheen should go. After that, apply your mattifying product, a product designed to absorb oil on the face, if you do not want shine." Peter Thomas Roth

Safety in Numbers

"I always recommend an SPF of 30, but I wouldn't leave the house without at least an SPF 15." June Jacobs

Souped-Up Sunscreen

"Look for multiple ingredients in your broad-spectrum sunscreen. You need A and B blockers. Look for an SPF 30 with physical and chemical sunscreens. There is very rarely one thing that does it all in nature. Everything is a complex biosynthetic event. Biology is all about interactions. Ingredients like Parsol 1789 and Mexoryl are great, but in combination with other products. It's like with cooking: don't spice a meal with one spice; use a combination." Dennis Gross, MD

Your "D" Dose

"It's a myth that you need to go out into the sun without sun protection to get your daily dose of vitamin D. You can absorb sunlight through the retina of the eye and you only need a minimal amount of exposure. Better yet, take a supplement!" Jan Marini

Got You Covered

"It is best to lock sunscreen or sunblock into your hairline and to coat the face and body evenly indoors before you hit the beach. Burn spots are derived from the incomplete application of a sun product, usually [when it's] applied in the sun where we often are already perspiring. This makes it difficult to get full body protection." Jim Miller

Who's on First

"Always apply sunscreen first, then allow it to absorb into the skin for at least three to five minutes before applying moisturizer." Giella

Turn Back the Sun

"Not using sun protection is the number-one mistake [women make]. The regular use of sunscreen with UVA protection is mandatory to reverse damage— you can't reverse until you begin to prevent—along with retinoids: tretinoin, tazarotene. Retinoids are also effective for acne [on women] of all ages. Use products on all sun-exposed areas. Avobenzone is good for only UVA rays, not UVB, so it must be in combo with an SPF B blocker. Everyone is looking forward to Mexoryl [a sunscreen used in Europe that is awaiting FDA approval], but zinc oxide and titanium dioxide are also very good. All antioxidants reduce UV damage by reducing the free radicals and enzymes activated by the sun's UV waves." Mary Lupo, MD

Sunscreen Reminder

"To prevent the hands and neck from revealing age, use sun protection and sunscreen. Also, active anti-aging products should be applied to those areas as well." Jeffrey Dover, MD

Eye Q

"If your sunscreen tends to burn your eyes when you sweat, apply a wax-based lip balm, such as Chapstick, around your eyes to prevent the sunscreen from migrating into them." Rick Noodleman, MD

Understanding the Lingo

"At SPF 12 and above, products are deemed to be sunblocks. While SPF 15 can block about ninety-four percent of the sun's burning rays, SPF 30 does a great job blocking ninety-seven-point-six percent of the rays. It is very difficult to claim that much more of the sun's burning rays can be blocked with higher 45–60 SPFs." Jim Miller

Sunscreen Selection

"There's a sunscreen that's right for you. The key is to test different formulas—gels, lotions, creams, waxes, et cetera, to see what works best. For drier skin, I recommend using Revercel's Oil-Free Sun Defense SPF 30+ daily for optimum full-spectrum protection. This light, non-greasy lotion is also perfect for wearing under makeup. For active people, try Revercel's Oil-Free Sun Defense Gel SPF 30, a lightweight, oil-free gel containing Parsol 1789 for optimum UVA protection and Octinoxate 7.5% for UVB protection. Waterproof and fragrance-free, it's great for active people with oily or acne-prone skin who spend time in the sun." Rick Noodleman, MD

Love Your Sunscreen

"In choosing a sunscreen, it is important that one selects a sunscreen that one likes. The texture, feel, and scent of the sunscreen is just as important as its effectiveness. Clearly, it is important to choose an SPF 15, 30, or 45 for the appropriate use, but if the individual doesn't like the feel, the texture, the scent, or the thickness of the product, they will not use it and the SPF will be of no use whatsoever. We like using both UVA and UVB screens in a single product to give broad-spectrum sunscreen protection. There are new sunscreens coming from Europe which have broader UVA protection than those available in America, but these are not FDA approved and not commercially available in this country. Spray-on sunscreens are terrific, but they must be applied regularly." Jeffrey Dover, MD

Sensitive Sunscreens

"If you are sensitive to chemical sunscreens, use sunscreens with physical blocking agents [i.e., titanium dioxide, zinc oxide] and wear protective clothing." Rick Noodleman, MD

Miracle Mist?

"It's hard to get even coverage [with a spray-on sunscreen]. There are going to be areas where you overlap and skip." Jessica Wu, MD

Key Ingredient

"Look for sun care with active ingredients like titanium dioxide, which reflects the sun's burning rays. I highly recommend this kind of sun care, especially if it is waterproof, sweatproof, oil-and-PABA free, and with UVA and UVB protection." Jim Miller

Sunscreen Specs

"Choose a broad-spectrum sunscreen that offers protection from both UVA and UVB rays with an SPF of at least 15." Rick Noodleman, MD

Wonder from Down Under

"In Australia, they have zinc oxide in very tiny particles. Instead of being white, it's transparent. It doesn't give you the pastiness. It's not approved in the U.S. yet." Jessica Wu, MD

Consistency Counts

"Apply your sunscreen frequently throughout the day, especially on the face, ears, neck, back of the neck, chest and hands, regardless of weather. Always reapply sunscreen after swimming or sweating." Rick Noodleman, MD

Multipurpose Performer

"Look for a sunscreen that contains antioxidants. Try to find an all-in-one product like a tinted moisturizer with SPF and antioxidants." Jessica Wu, MD

SUNLESS SOLUTIONS

The Buzz from the Beauty Editor

Self-tanners are a fabulous way to get a glow without the sun damage, but if you don't have the time and the patience, there are a few quicker ways to achieve similar results. One of my favorites is Jergens Natural Glow Daily Moisturizer, $5.99, which is essentially a self-tanner cut with plenty of body lotion, and designed for easy, daily application. I also love DuWop Revolution Tinted Body Moisturizer with SPF 15 and Shimmer, $21, which offers subtle color, shimmer, and sunscreen in one easy product. For more color and coverage, try one of the new spray-on "stockings," like Sally Hansen Airbrush Legs, $10, or Air Stocking, $28. Spray-on stockings let you skip the real thing, without exposing pasty-white winter legs.

Insider Information from the Beauty Bunch

Face Tips

"Apply a light, oil-free moisturizing lotion before self-tanner. The self-tanners that are designed for the face do have a more refined molecule, so you will get a little heavier pigment from them. Rinse it off after it's processed, about six hours later, because your pores show the little dots. If you wash it off, you won't look so spotted." Angela Nice

Sunless Strategy

"When using a self-tanner, scrub first to exfoliate and even out the dead skin cells, and then apply evenly. Wash hands immediately, for they will stain really dark, or use rubber gloves. Avoid knees and elbows; they will also stain very dark. Start with more subtle color; for darker color, apply it twice. To maintain your new tan, reapply every three days. My Natural Looking Self Tanner is fragrance-free and has a very natural color." Peter Thomas Roth

Shade Shopping

"A person should not have to rely on a 'shade' of self-tanner to match their skintone. Fake Bake is formulated to transform even the palest of skintones into a beautiful bronze color. If they desire a much deeper tan, we encourage them to reapply three consecutive nights to achieve optimum results." Clarissa Azar

Eliminating the Odor

"There is nothing you can do to eliminate the smell. It's the gas that's being released from your pores. The chemical exchange is what you smell. Wait six hours for the tan to process, then shower or mask it with perfume. All self-tanners do it. It's not the product; it's actually your own body causing the odor." Angela Nice

Spray-Tan Stealer

"A hot tub is the fastest way to kill a spray-on tan. Take a dip in the Jacuzzi or a hot bath if you have streaky lines you want to get rid of, but if you like your canned tan, avoid soaking in hot water." Kathryn Alice

Trouble Spots

"Apply a moisturizing product [to spots that tend to get darker, like knees, elbows, et cetera], like the dry oil from Fake Bake, to prevent too much absorption of the tanning product while still allowing enough of the tanning agents to penetrate to give color to those areas. Fair skin benefits from applying all-over body moisturizer prior to self-tanning for a diluted approach." Clarissa Azar

Magical Muscle Tone

"You can fake muscle tone with an airbrush tan more easily than with a self-applied tanner. The main thing is to look at yourself in overhead light, and pay attention to where your shadowing is naturally. Apply extra self-tanner to those shaded areas, like the obliques of the stomach, the inner and outer thighs, the panty line, and the tops of the shoulders. This will give you a little more of an elongated look." Angela Nice

Banish Brown Dots

"Many people experience little brown dots forming in the pores of their bikini line after an application of sunless tanner. These brown dots come from the tint in their sunless-tanning product, and they can be avoided. Gently dab a very light layer of lotion onto the bikini line area before self-tanning to help prevent the overabsorption of tint into the pores." Fiona Locke

Find Your Formula

"Airbrush tanning utilizes a 'full-strength' dose of self-tanner with 'sticking power.' This liquid form of Fake Bake is a concentrate, and it's best when used by a professional. A gel, like Fake Bake Xtreme gel, is the next [most] concentrated form, with less moisture to provide a quick-dry approach, and a much deeper, darker color guide for quicker results. It's for the person who wants to out-tan everyone.

Our lotion has a fifty-percent longer life on the skin than any other self-tanner. The moisture content also aids in longevity. It's our most popular formula, and blended in a way that fits all skin types and tones. Our mousse is a diluted version of the others, creating a much lighter dose of bronzing. It dries quickly and glides on a much lighter color at the onset. If the client is new with self-tanners, then we recommend trying the mousse first and then graduating to deeper, more concentrated options." Clarissa Azar

Maintaining Your Glow

"Don't exfoliate [after tanning]. Keep skin moisturized. We sell self-tanner to be used as touch-ups for the spray tanning. We also do a treatment called a vacation tan, with treatments three days in a row. The first day, we exfoliate and airbrush tan, followed by another airbrush tan, then another. We have had people say it lasts three weeks. People can do this at home, too. I do think it's good to get the old tan off in between, but there are some people who are always self-tanned. If you let it fade and exfoliate completely in between, and let the color get all the way down, you will have a more even tan. Otherwise, it can look freckly in spots." Angela Nice

The Tinted Advantage

"You have the ability to see where you are applying the tan when you have a color guide in the product. We coined a phrase for our product back in 1996 that says it is a 'shows-where-it-goes' formula. A white or clear self-tanner can be a nightmare because by the time your tan develops it is too late to undo your mistakes. You just pray the phone doesn't ring mid-application with these products!" Clarissa Azar

Stop the Staining

"Avoid stains on hands and feet from the use of self-tanners by exfoliating and creating a barrier. The skin on the hands and feet is very porous and just loves to suck up sunless tanners. Prior to the application of a self-tanner, whether at home or professionally, spend a little extra time in the shower scrubbing the heels and balls of feet with a pumice stone to reduce calloused areas and remove excess dead skin. Also, make sure to moisturize the bottoms of the feet so they won't be so thirsty. Always apply self-tanner carefully and in circular motions, and wash hands afterwards. You may choose to wear latex gloves to keep hands stain-free when self-tanning at home. If you're receiving a professional sunless treatment, the technician will apply a barrier cream to your hands and feet to keep them free of staining. Be aware that nails will also stain, so you want to carefully avoid applying self-tanner to the toenails, and carefully wash fingernails with a nail brush over the top of the nails and underneath. A coat of nail polish also does the trick to keep staining away." Fiona Locke

The Tinted Advantage

"The advantage of using a tinted self-tanner is to enjoy a beautiful tan minus the streaks and blotches. We recommend wearing gloves—enclosed with our product line—so that you can take your time and apply the product evenly. This also eliminates 'tanning' your palms. When you are finished applying tanner to the body, remove the gloves and smooth product onto the back of the hands using a makeup sponge." Clarissa Azar

Residual Issues

"Skin is a great sponge that will retain any residue that is left on it. For the most even tan, always use an exfoliator that will not leave any soap on the skin. Even if you think you have rinsed thoroughly, soap can still be an issue. That is why we have created our exfoliators without soap, so that the tan will go on evenly and will fade evenly as well." Clarissa Azar

Step-by-Step Self-Tanner

1. **Make it foolproof:** "Wear rubber gloves. That's the number-one thing. You want to massage that tanner into the pores. Buy a box of medical gloves. Tan your hands last."

2. **Pick the right shade:** "Most people reach for dark. I usually tell them to start with medium, and then you can always layer it. You will typically get results from any of the colors unless you have a really dark skin-tone. In our spa, we only use light or medium. A second application makes it last a little longer. A lot of people are happy when they start with the light, and it's just perfect. It's just enough. The difference between tinted self-tanners and clear ones is that the tinted kind offers a color guide for blending, so that you can see if you missed a spot, or if you haven't rubbed it in well. The shower will rinse off the residue, and there's instant gratification. You can run to the pool and hang out there, though it would be kind of a bummer if you were to jump into the pool."

3. **Pick the right formula:** "Sprays or mists let you get to hard-to-reach areas, and you can tip the can upside down. Their main advantage is that they really let you cover the back and the back of your legs. But you still have to massage them in, and a lot of people don't do that. They think they can just coat themselves and not have to blend, but you do have to blend it in. We learned the hard way on that one. That's how you get streaks. Creams are

typically better for drier skins, and gels for oilier skins. Gel is less sticky, but I feel you get the best penetration with a cream. You usually get a more uniform result."

4. **Exfoliate:** "If all else fails, use a washcloth. It goes a long way. Really, really exfoliate yourself with it. There are so many scrubs, and they all will do the trick. Even taking your towel and drying yourself off very well will work really well. Then open the bathroom door and let the steam out. It's nice to have a resting period before you apply your self-tanner, because your pores are filled with moisture from the shower, and the product won't penetrate as much. Allow a cool-down period, particularly for perspiration-prone areas like under breasts or arms. Water and self-tanner don't mix too well; it leads to streaking."

5. **Prep:** "A little lotion can prevent areas like knees and elbows from getting too dark. Use some on knees, elbows, ankles, knuckles of hands and feet, and in between the webbing of the toes. Also put lotion on the cuticles of the toes and covering the nail bed. It feels good and it's good for your nails to have that lotion on. For a salon spray tan, you need to apply this. Also put lotion heavily on the bottoms of the feet so that soles don't absorb it, or use a fresh mat. Wrap hair in a towel, pin it back, or use a shower cap. Get your hair out of the way so you can see yourself completely. Hair doesn't usually take to self-tanner, because it doesn't produce the same chemical reaction, but I still don't like to expose my color to it or have the smell on my hair."

6. **Apply:** "Massage your self-tanner in with the gloves on, even with a salon spray tan. I like to blend it all in and then pat dry any excess, but typically you can blend it all in because it's such a fine spray and it's very absorbent. Don't forget to apply under the breasts. We often don't lift them up high enough or the client sweats it all off. Another trouble spot is the underarms. Some women forget the underarms, or the self-tanner didn't mix right with their antiperspirant so it didn't take. Don't put self-tanner on the bottoms of your feet. You don't tan there. You should never do that. It also won't take evenly."

7. **Hands off:** "One of the biggest mistakes people make is touching themselves after putting it on. That's a big no-no. It gets all over palms, in nails, cuticles. It's just an obvious sign that you have got self-tanner on, and it's hard to get it off fingertips. Even though it's massaged in, when you scrub and itch and your hands are sweaty, you pull tanning solution off skin and onto hands. Wash your hands three times if you've touched yourself when you have self-tanner on. *Really* wash them." Angela Nice

Muddy Mistake

"[The biggest mistake is] lack of exfoliation and care for specific areas of the body, such as ankles, elbows, and heels, therefore resulting in a dirty, dark residue where the product can only sit on the surface." Clarissa Azar

Making Muscles

"A professional should be consulted [if you want to apply self-tanner to enhance the look of muscles]. Typically, a makeup artist is well-seasoned with these techniques and uses airbrushing to accomplish this by shading appropriate areas of the body to define muscle tone. Meanwhile, you can use a bronzer, like Fake Bake Beyond Bronze Convertible bronzing blush, to 'highlight' areas of your body or face, giving a more pronounced glow just where you want it." Clarissa Azar

Scent Reduction

To minimize the odor of self-tanning "choose a self-tanner free of harsh chemicals. Upon completion of application, you can lightly brush over the skin with a clean, dry towel, which aids in reducing the immediate scent." Clarissa Azar

Face Fix

"Use a makeup sponge if you desire a lighter appearance on the face." Clarissa Azar

Back It Up

"Women find the back to be the hardest area for them to reach. We encourage them to purchase a back brush, which is a spa tool that has a sponge on the end, to help out." Clarissa Azar

UNDOING THE DAMAGE

The Buzz from the Beauty Editor

Already sporting the telltale signs of sun damage? All is not lost. Dermatologists can do more than ever before to reverse existing damage, and many of the newest topicals and treatments are suitable for all skintones and skin types. I have medium-tan olive skin, so I've always been wary of lasers, because the only thing worse than having brown spots is having white spots from lack of pigment. Fortunately, some of the newer lasers are safe for even the darkest skintones.

Insider Information from the Beauty Bunch

Reversing Sun Damage

"One of the newest [methods for reversing sun damage] is the Fraxel laser. This type of laser helps to fade brown spots and blotchiness as well as soften fine lines, with very little recovery time. It works on all skin types and colors. That's what's different about this laser compared to all the other lasers that have preceded it, because the other lasers have been limited to fair skintones. This works by heating up the collagen in tiny little dots, so instead of burning off the whole layer of skin, you leave the skin between the microscopic dots and it heals faster. It doesn't burn off the epidermis; it goes deeper so that it tightens the skin without risk of scarring and discoloration. It's a very new laser, and no one knows how long the results will last, but it is very promising. But what we've been doing for several years with great results is IPL [intense pulsed light, or photofacial]. It is increasingly popular in my practice, and there's very little recovery time, but it's not appropriate for very dark skintones. To treat and prevent sun damage, you need a very good homecare routine as well. You can't come in for a monthly photofacial and in between go bake in the sun. It's a waste of everybody's time. I have a patient who is a young woman in her early thirties who had baked in the sun since she was twelve. She had sun damage, freckles, and lines. We did six photofacials and she looked six to seven years younger, but one weekend on top of a mountain for a ski trip and all of the freckles came back. So we had to start all over." Jessica Wu, MD

Treating Sun Damage

"There are a variety of options available. I like to divide them into prevention, topical treatments, and laser- or light-based procedures. The most important way to reverse sun damage is sun avoidance, sun protection, use of effective sunscreen, and appropriate clothing and hats. I recommend sun-screening year-round with a minimum of SPF 15 from October fifteenth to April fifteenth in the Northeast and the Northwest and less sunny climes, and an SPF 30 or higher in the rest of the country year-round and in [less sunny] geographic areas from April fifteenth until October fifteenth. When actively pursuing sun activities, it is best to use an SPF 30 or 45, a hat, and protective clothing, and to reapply sunscreen every two to three hours. Effective topical treatments include topical retinoids (vitamin-A derivatives), topical vitamins, topical botanicals, and topical growth factors. The FDA-approved retinoids used predominately in this country are Retin-A, Renova, Avage, and Differin. They all work relatively similarly. Avage is the best for its speed of action and its effectiveness for dyspigmentation. For those who do not have dyspigmentation, I like to prescribe either Renova for those who prefer creamy products or Retin-A Micro Gel for those who prefer less-creamy products." Jeffrey Dover, MD

Vitamin Power

"Wear topical vitamin C to boost the effectiveness of your sunscreen. I recommend Revercel's Vita-C Infusion, an oil-free, lightweight, powerful antioxidant powder-cream containing L-ascorbic acid to protect and repair the skin and prevent environmental damage. It softens the appearance of fine lines and wrinkles that may be unresponsive to other anti-aging products." Rick Noodleman, MD

THE PRODUCT FILES

Sunscreens

The Buzz from the Beauty Editor

The key to ensuring that your skin is protected is to look for broad- or full-spectrum protection, and don't trust the marketing: if it doesn't say titanium dioxide, zinc oxide, or Parsol 1789 on the active ingredient list, then it doesn't shield you from UVB rays and should be avoided. (UVB rays lead to skin cancer; UVA rays cause aging and the hyperpigmentation and wrinkles that accompany it.) Give sunscreen a few moments to sink in before continuing your skin-care routine. I'm not that particular about body sunscreens, as long as they offer broad-spectrum protection, but my facial sunscreens are part of my skincare routine, so they need to be light, sheer, and moisturizing without being greasy. My favorites are June Jacobs Spa Collection Oil-Free Sunscreen Mist SPF 15, $32, Shiseido Ultimate Sun Protection Lotion SPF 55, $37, Jan Marini Antioxidant Daily Face Protection SPF 30, $40, and Neutrogena UltraSheer Dry-Touch Sunblock SPF 45, $10.

What the Pros Choose

The experts' recommendations led me to discover several fabulous products, including a couple I never knew existed. I wasn't surprised to see that June Jacobs, Peter Thomas Roth, Jim Miller, and Meg Thompson all pick their own formulas; their sunscreens are among the best on the market. Thompson specifies her Madge Cosmetics Madgic Moisture SPF 15 with shimmer. Danielle Browning also picks Peter Thomas Roth, specifically his Max Sheer All Day Moisture Defense Lotion with SPF 30, as well as Sonya Dakar 365 SPF 30, as her favorites. Others are fresh picks: Leaf & Rusher (Julie Hewett), Epione Total Block 60 (Meredith Green), Catherine Atzen Ultra Preventive Sunblock SPF 30 (Vanessa Talabac), and The Vital Image Sunshield Moisturizer (Linda Deslauriers). Neutrogena is the choice of Hara Glick and Wende Zomnir (Active Dry Touch SPF 45). Zomnir also loves the hard-to-find sunscreens from French giant La Roche Posay. Charles Worthington loves Sisley Body Sun Cream; Shauna Raisch likes Aveda Dual Nature Face Protection SPF 15; Dee DeLuca-Mattos picks Clarins SPF 15; Debra Luftman picks MDForte SPF 30, and Gabrielle Ophals likes SkinCeuticals Daily Sun Defense SPF 20. Shan Albert makes the most unusual choice: she counts on mineral makeup, such as Colorescience, which has an SPF 20. "It's water-resistant; does not run while perspiring, therefore does not sting the eyes; and at the same time that it is protecting you from the sun it makes the skin look fabulous. Men can wear it because it doesn't look like makeup and I've used Colorescience on my grandbabies with great success—no allergic reaction and no sunburns."

Sunless Tanners

The Buzz from the Beauty Editor

I cheated in this category. Since my skin is naturally olive and tanned, I used my husband as a guinea pig for some of these products. The other recommendations came about through friends. In case you haven't already heard, before applying self-tanner, exfoliate, exfoliate, exfoliate. And go easy on naturally darker parts, like knees and elbows. Another tip is to mix a little facial self-tanner in with your morning moisturizer, and make it part of your daily routine. The moisturizer cuts the self-tanner, making it goofproof. My favorites are Fake Bake Sunless Self-Tanning Lotion, $22.95, and Tan Towels, $20.

What the Pros Choose

Again, I learned something here. As expected, Jim Miller, June Jacobs, and Peter Thomas Roth all pick their own exceptional products. Other bestselling picks include SkinCeuticals Sans Soleil (Debra Luftman), Lancôme Mousse (Wende Zomnir), Aveda Sun Source (Shauna Raisch), Clarins (Hara Glick), and California Tan Sunless Self Tanner Tinted Foam (Fiona Locke). St. Tropez Whipped Bronze Instant Self-Tanning Mousse is the product of choice for Charles Worthington, while Gabrielle Ophals likes St. Tropez Tinted Self-Tanning Lotion because "it's brown, so you can see where you've applied it." Vanessa Talabac picks Catherine Atzen Self Tanning Lotion. Other winners: SUN, picked by Julie Hewett and Dee DeLuca-Mattos; Magic Tan, the choice of Meredith Green; Mystic Tan, Meg Thompson's choice; and Fake Bake, Clarissa Azar's pick. Dee DeLuca-Mattos also specifies a facial self-tanner, Jergens Natural Glow Daily Moisturizer, and raves, "It builds color each time you apply it. It's the best."

Chapter Nine

Healthy Hair Care:
Treat Your Tresses to Headturning Style

When you have as much hair as I do, a bad hair day is nearly impossible to conceal. A hat would be handy, but when my hair is at its most frizzy and fried, it's nearly impossible to coax a cloche over my curls. That's why, like most women, I'm obsessed with avoiding bad hair days. I buy hair products by the truckload, enlist any expert who'll listen for advice, and scan images of supermodels for the singular style that will change my life. Why the ardent interest in taming my tresses? Ask any woman the same question, and she'll tell you that her hair, more than any other single element of her look, has the ability to affect her mood and define her day. That's why I've devoted so much space to hair in this chapter and the next. On these pages, you'll learn how to style and smooth, how to wear it curly or straight, and how to communicate with your stylist to get the look you want.

THE *Beauty Bunch* BREAKDOWN

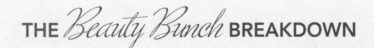

Nathaniel Hawkins: top New York City hairstylist whose celebrity fans include Winona Ryder, Gisele Bündchen, Heidi Klum, Kelly Ripa, Maggie Gyllenhaal, Marcia Cross, and Hilary Duff.

Linda Deslauriers: founder of Hair Garden, a holistic hair company based in Hawaii and Los Angeles, and the author of an upcoming hair-care book.

Barry Reitman: star hairstylist with over twenty-five years of experience serving an exclusive clientele of celebrities and royalty.

Michael O'Rourke: founder and master hairstylist of Sexy Hair Concepts.

Shauna Raisch: founder and owner of Twiggs Salonspa of Wayzata, a 3,700-square-foot high-end facility in the Twin Cities.

Jerome Lordet: star stylist at NYC's Pierre Michel Salon, his work has graced the heads of celebs like Sandra Bullock and Rebecca Gayheart.

Rachel Lindy: stylist at Los Angeles's Trim Salon and winner of *Allure*'s coveted Up and Coming Star Stylist award.

David Cotteblanche: star stylist and co-owner of New York City's Red Market Salon and Lounge in the trendy Meatpacking District.

Diane Gardner: Hollywood hairstylist, colorist, and makeup artist known as the Makeover Specialist.

Fabrice Gili: hair designer at Frédéric Fekkai Salon & Spa.

Jessica Tingley: hair designer at Frédéric Fekkai Salon & Spa in Beverly Hills, her work has graced celebrities such as Daisy Fuentes, Maggie Gyllenhaal, Mischa Barton, and Kerry Washington.

Damien Miano: celebrity hairstylist whose work has appeared in countless top magazines, including *Cosmopolitan*, *Glamour*, and *W*. Miano is co-owner of New York City's hot Miano Viél Salon.

Peter Lamas: founder and chairman of Lamas Beauty International, a rapidly growing, well-respected natural beauty–product manufacturer.

Charles Worthington: co-owner and creative director of Charles Worthington salons, with five locations in London and one in New York City, which attract celebrities like Mena Suvari and Jennifer Love Hewitt.

Jimmy Vanegas: founder and owner of Beauty Now Management.

Ouidad: stylist, salon owner, educator, and author who has earned a respected reputation as the Curly Hair Expert.

Fabien Roussel: top New York City stylist with the Julien Farel Salon whose work has appeared in *Allure*, *Bride's*, *Elle Décor*, *Glamour*, and *Harper's Bazaar*.

Kattia Solano: owner of the hip Butterfly Studio in New York City, which has been featured in Daily Candy and *Allure*.

HAIR CARE

The Buzz from the Beauty Editor

With my long, thick, curly hair, hair care plays a major role in my life. I devote almost as much time to thinking about my hair as I do to actually caring for it. I say I wash it every other day, but if it still looks good or if I'm not going anywhere, I might stretch it out a third day. I need to hold on to as much moisture as I can get. I use so many products that occasionally I have to use a vinegar rinse to remove excess buildup. My hair is left silky-smooth and soft.

Insider Information from the Beauty Bunch

Cider Rules

"Organic unfiltered apple-cider vinegar has a cleansing and stimulating function on the scalp. It also helps with dandruff, itchiness, and hair thinning. You can apply it directly onto the scalp with a cotton ball or as a rinse. Leave it on for at least thirty minutes." Linda Deslauriers

Natural Selection

"I don't think that there is a single product line that has the best of everything; I pick and choose products from different lines. To pick a product, I look for a reputable company first, and then I smell it. For women, it's all about lotions and potions. If it smells good, they will love it. When you see women looking at products, nine times out of ten they will unscrew the cap and smell them. So I go by the smell first, and then I see what the product can do." Barry Reitman

Feed Your Head

"Eat green for your scalp and hair! Green vegetables, algae, and fruit are excellent sources of important vitamins and trace elements." Linda Deslauriers

Cool Idea

"Try to rinse your hair with cold water. It closes the cuticle and smoothes the hair. If [the cuticle] is open, it absorbs heat and pollutants. And protect it from the sun. Use some sort of screen on it or cover it up." Michael O'Rourke

Hair Hope

"There is no reason for anyone's hair not to look brilliant. If your hair looks fabulous, it's working. If not, it's time for a new prescription." Barry Reitman

Salt Your Scalp

"Celtic sea salt supplies the body, scalp, and hair with over eighty trace elements. Use it for cooking and on your salad and take a tiny pinch daily, especially when experiencing hair loss." Linda Deslauriers

Mane Maintenance

If you are in dire need of a highlight or color, but your appointment is a week away, Shauna Raisch offers this advice: "Wear a hat and prebook your next appointment before you leave the salon." And for maintaining a great cut and color? "Begin with a great haircut and make sure you have the right products at home to work with it. Using the right products will keep your hair in optimal condition, and don't forget to retouch color on a regular basis."

Shirk Your Shampoo

"Shampoo less. Dilute your shampoo with water. Skip a day. This avoids drying your hair out and gives oily hair a chance to get back into balance. Rotate shampoos. Every time you wash your hair use a different shampoo, which means you have at least two bottles in your bathroom. This strengthens your scalp's immunity towards one product." Linda Deslauriers

Mix It Up

"You should alternate shampoos and conditioners daily. One day, use one set, and the next, use another set. This will help your hair stay healthy, and it won't get used to one product." Jerome Lordet

Cool Condition

"After washing your shampoo out with warm water, rinse hair with cold water. This will close the cuticle layer, which protects the hair shaft, and it provides a smooth surface for the light to reflect, resulting in shinier hair. It also creates more volume because each individual hair stands up more once the cold water firms up the tissue surrounding it. Once you are used to rinsing your hair with cold water in the shower, expand this invigorating habit to your whole body." Linda Deslauriers

Shampoo Schedule

"It's better to shampoo hair less often than more often, about every other day. Especially if you use a blow-dryer, you really should make it last a couple of days." Rachel Lindy

Free Your Mind

"The scalp has among the largest pores of the body. The body uses it to eliminate toxins. Anthony Morrocco's Zen Detox assists this process greatly." Linda Deslauriers

Put Away Your Products

"Try a product fast. Reduce your consumption of body care products to a bare minimum. Try an all-purpose product, like the Anthony Morrocco Method shampoos that you can use on your hair, face, body, and even for shaving. Don't use any commercial styling products for a week and see if you can survive. The goal is to give your body a rest and to gain independence." Linda Deslauriers

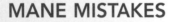

MANE MISTAKES

The Buzz from the Beauty Editor

I've made many mistakes with my hair. In the eighties, I straightened my naturally curly hair and wore it hard and helmetlike. It was unflattering, frumpy, and most of all aging, but looking older was not a concern at sixteen. Most of the mistakes mentioned by the pros are made by women who, like me, are fighting the hair that God gave them. Battling nature is time-consuming and costly, and it makes you a slave to your hair, so embrace your hair's natural texture and make the most of it.

Insider Information from the Beauty Bunch

Look Letdown

"[A common mistake] is when you see that the style doesn't work with the client. It's a total look. Some haircuts are nice, but they're not working for the person. It's about proportion, which is very important for the face. Or I see too many layers." David Cotteblanche

Fighting Nature

"It's strange. It doesn't matter what hair they're born with—they think it's problem hair, whether it's fine and thinning or thick and curly. A stylist needs to make you realize that you are blessed. It's how you handle that hair at that time, whatever hair you have. It's not going to be changed. This is mine. I love it. What can I do to make it look cool? You just have to know how to handle it and handle it right." Michael O'Rourke

Faulty Colors

"One of the biggest mistakes I see is when women have the wrong hair color for their coloring, the wrong tone for their skin and eye color. They are stuck on whatever they first tried. Another mistake is a haircut that suits their lifestyle, but not their face. They leave it long so that they can clip it up or chop it off because it's convenient or cut bangs because they are easier, with no consideration of their facial features. Many women choose styles that are easy to care for but that don't [suit them]." Diane Gardner

Lengthy Errors

"The number-one mistake that I see is the wrong hair length, when the length does not really pay attention to the face shape. The first thing you see in a haircut is not the layers or the texturizing, but the length. If it doesn't work, it's the length. Either it's too short, too long, or too angled. There are three major face shapes. The oval face works with every hair length. With a long face, avoid hair that is all one length. Break it up with layers. With a round face shape, you have to be really careful to not make the hair too round. It's important that the cut has some angles. When you don't have any layers, it emphasizes roundness. A cut that is all one length does not frame the face to cut this roundness. Some women have square faces, and with this shape, you have to be really careful to not make the hair too bobbish-looking, which emphasizes squareness. You need something softer, with more length and width. It's also important to take the shape of the neck into consideration. Shorter hair looks good on necks that aren't too long. If the hair is too short, it makes the neck appear longer, so you want something in between if your neck is long. If you have no neck, wear the hair as short as possible to open up the neck. When you look at the face, you should look all the way down to the collarbone. The neck is where it all starts." Fabrice Gili

Natural Woman

"Everybody tries to reverse the texture that they have. If you have curly hair, leave it curly. Don't damage your natural hair. It's easier. If you are going

against the nature of your hair, it's very difficult." David Cotteblanche

Style Stumbles

"A lot of people glop product on the top of their head, and don't distribute it all the way through, because they're in a hurry. Another mistake is to style hair in sections that are too big. Or they ignore the back. The front looks perfect, but the back is all frizzy." Jessica Tingley

Lazy Locks

"The biggest [offender] is the clip in the hair, holding it all back. The guy with the ponytail and the woman with the big clippie should be knocked off by the beauty police. What it says is that they don't care. The truth is that they do care, but they are not thinking about it. For millions of women, the clippie is the statement that they don't care or are lazy. If you are pulling your hair back all the time, then you don't have a defined haircut." Diane Gardner

Styling Error

"Trying too hard. They try too hard or don't do enough. It's both. Women take a very negative position and blame themselves for not being able to do their own hair, when very often it is the haircut speaking and not the client's ability. Your hair should not be that big of an ordeal unless you have an inordinate amount of hair. Hedgehog hair can be understandably difficult to style, but you can facilitate it being better or easier to style. When you try too hard, it looks forced, not natural." Damien Miano

Over-Dry

"A common styling mistake that women make is drying their hair too long, with the heat on too high. They overdry it, which damages the hair very quickly.

Another mistake is not using the right tools, the right dryer, or the right brush." Fabrice Gili

TRIM TIMELINE

The Buzz from the Beauty Editor

I once went one year and three months without a haircut, because I couldn't make it to New York City to see the one stylist who can cut my curls properly. A good haircut is that important. I don't recommend trying this yourself, however. I endured six long months of hair hatred before that long-awaited haircut. But how long should you wait between haircuts? It depends on the length. Short hair can only go for short periods of time, like a few weeks, between cuts, whereas long hair can go longer. Ask your stylist, and prebook your next appointment before you leave the salon.

Insider Information from the Beauty Bunch

Cut Frequency

"I wouldn't recommend any longer than two to three months for a trim." Peter Lamas

Time to Tame

"The maximum you should let your hair go between cuts is eight weeks, whether you are maintaining your length or letting it grow. A stylist can take off just the ends, so that your hair is healthy and the ends are not thin or split." Barry Reitman

Cut Frequency

"If you have a very edgy, very fashionable haircut, then [get a cut every] three to four weeks, because it requires more maintenance." David Cotteblanche

Cut Often

"If you want to maintain a shorter cut, and not add any length, then a cut every four weeks will keep it crisp and perfect. Otherwise, you can go six to eight weeks, and on the longer side for long hair." Jessica Tingley

CATASTROPHIC CUTS

The Buzz from the Beauty Editor

The worst cut I ever had happened when I was sixteen years old, and it was so cataclysmic that it took my hair four years to recover. The stylist essentially parted my hair from ear to ear, and shaved the entire lower half of my hair off. This made pulling it into a ponytail impossible, and as my hair grew out, it pushed out the top layer of hair, creating an unfortunate ledge. How could I let such a tragedy befall my hair? I believed the (inexperienced) stylist when he said that the cut would thin out my hair and make it more manageable. And even though I had serious doubts, I was too shy to speak up. Fortunately, most bad haircuts are not so horrific. Stylists cite choppy, unblended 'dos and boring, suburban styles at the top of their "worst cut" lists.

Insider Information from the Beauty Bunch

Tress Neglect

"The biggest mistake women make with their hair is not being consistent with their salon appointments. The issue with that is that things change, your hair condition changes, and your stylist needs to make sure you are still doing what is right for your hair, even if you are letting it grow. The other mistake that women make is choosing the wrong hair color. Either they pick the wrong color, one that doesn't enhance their natural beauty, or, even if they've been warned, they are shocked at the maintenance required to keep up their color." Barry Reitman

Bad-Cut Lowdown

"Bad layers are chunky and don't blend in with the other pieces of hair. No matter how you move your hair, it falls in chunks." Jessica Tingley

Un-Blendable

"The most offensive haircuts are those that don't blend. Layers are cut into the hair, and there's no relation to the rest of the hair. Or there is some height cut in the crown with short layers, and there's no relation to the rest of the cut. It may not be as bad as a mullet, and the stylist can style it so that it looks sleek and it works, but when you get it home you can't work with it. It's a bad haircut. It doesn't look blended and the lines don't flow. Another bad haircut is one that's boring. A lot of suburban haircuts are not bad; they're just boring. It's easy to take a woman and just give her a one-length haircut, and it very rarely looks great on everyone or every type of hair. A boring haircut is almost as bad to me as a bad haircut, because it's something that doesn't take advantage of the natural texture of the hair and doesn't flatter. But unblended cuts are my pet peeve." Damien Miano

Frequent Flubs

"The most common mistake I see in haircuts is when the client/stylist is cutting for a trend, rather than for the client's hair/facial structure/age. If you're noticing the hair and not the person, it's a bad cut. The most common mistake women make is trying to pull off a style that isn't right for their face, lifestyle, and, most importantly, age." Peter Lamas

QUICK STYLES

The Buzz from the Beauty Editor

While the stylists disagreed on some things, they were universal in their support of low-maintenance hair. They unanimously agreed that, with a good haircut, a morning routine should be fairly quick and simple.

Insider Information from the Beauty Bunch

Morning Commitment

"[It should take a woman] ten minutes [to do her hair in the morning]. Unless your hair is really thick, and then twenty minutes. Longer than that, and there is something wrong with your haircut." Damien Miano

Timely Tresses

"How long it takes to do your hair depends on your hair type. You may have the kind of cut that you shake out and blow-dry and that's wonderful, but you may not have that kind of hair type. You need to spend the correct amount of time if your schedule allows it.

It's truly about your lifestyle, because that dictates how much time you have to spend on your hair." Michael O'Rourke

Speedy Style

"If your hair is cut correctly, it will fall right into place, and will be easy to style. I'm more of a shower, shampoo, and let your hair air-dry type of stylist. If your hairdresser spends an hour fooling with your hair to make it look good, you'll take two hours to achieve the same result. I just can't see how anyone should spend more then fifteen minutes on their hair." Peter Lamas

Quick Fix

"If you're spending more than thirty minutes on your hair, it's too elaborate. You shouldn't be spending that much time on it, and you shouldn't be struggling with anything. Otherwise, you have the wrong cut." Jessica Tingley

Sensible Styling

"Don't leave a salon without a style that you can easily do at home. It shouldn't take you more than fifteen to twenty minutes." Barry Reitman

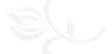

CLASSIC CUTS

The Buzz from the Beauty Editor

A great haircut should take several things into account: your hair's natural texture, your face shape, your personality. And it should fall right into place when it's wet.

Insider Information from the Beauty Bunch

Celeb Speak

"I like the new shorter trend. Jessica Simpson had a shorter style on the cover of *Elle*. It has some long angles in the front. It's fantastic. That's what's coming up [right now]. For three to four years, all we saw was long hair. Now, there is a trend toward shorter hair. It's more chic, more elegant, but still sexy. At a Chanel party, Ivanka Trump had cut her hair a little shorter than a bob. It looked great." David Cotteblanche

Personal Style

"I think haircuts are very, very personal. It comes down to the type of hair. You have to look at the hair. Fine hair shouldn't be layered to death. It should be cut more bluntly, so you leave some more hair. It encourages the look of full hair but doesn't become overpowering. With thick hair, some of the weight should be taken out on the inside so that the client is dealing with less hair and it's not so difficult to manage. A stylist should also take into account the face shape and the personality." Michael O'Rourke

Fine Cut

"Fine, limp hair should be cut above the collarbone for volume, with long layers to give it some movement. Anything longer gets stringy-looking." Jessica Tingley

Face Framing

"One general rule of thumb with haircuts is to think of your hair as framing your face. If you hold one hand above your face and one hand below your face, and find your eyes as the center, it will look as if your face is in a frame and your hands are the top and bottom of the frame. Your hair should be as high as the top hand, and as long or short as the bottom hand,

and then your face is perfectly framed. It can be exaggerated; for example, you can wear it high on top with curls or teasing on the crown. Even if you wear your hair super long, give it a lot of volume on the top to balance it out, so that your eyes are the focus. Long hair just drags the eye down so that that no one is looking at your eyes; your hair is dragging you down and all they see is hair. So definitely frame your face, with your eyes as the center." Diane Gardner

Shape Shifting

"Oval and round face shapes are usually the easiest to deal with because they are softer. Triangular or rectangular face shapes should be very careful to be soft in the length and the layering. A pointy face or chin is the hardest face shape to deal with." Fabrice Gili

Ship Shape

"This is how I look at a haircut. If you wash it and shake it out, it should already have a shape, before you blow-dry it. It should show that lovely shape. Otherwise, something is wrong. If you are feeling uncomfortable, something is wrong. You should love that haircut before you even blow-dry it. It should start looking pretty. If you can't see the shape, how are you going to blow-dry it?" Michael O'Rourke

Short Chic

"If you look back, historically, Hollywood legends have always had short hair. It's been set and curled on top, but they all had shorter hair; every one of them. Even today. Think of Annette Bening, or Halle Berry's hair when it was short. That's my theory and I'm sticking to it." Diane Gardner

Youthful Hair

"You definitely want to go with a style suitable to your face shape, one that softens rather than creates contrast. Contrast will emphasize lines and signs of aging. The same goes for color; always work with lights and darks suitable to your face shape to create softness, not harshness. There are certain styles suitable to specific face shapes. Oval is the perfectly balanced face shape. Almost anything goes with the balance of this face. Round and square face shapes are similar in that both require creating narrowness through the sides of the face, the difference being that round faces should sport more angles and square faces should have more rounded softer lines. Pear-shaped faces need to add width through the forehead and decrease width through the chin area. Diamond face shapes need to add width through the forehead and the chin but need to decrease width through the cheek area. Oblong faces should decrease length of face and add width through the sides of the face. Heart-shaped faces need to decrease width through the forehead and add width through the chin area. Remember that for color, light increases width, and dark decreases width." Shauna Raisch

Cool Cuts

"A great haircut is fun and hair grows back. Now women are more willing to cut their hair than ever before. All the stars are cutting their hair. The young generation of actresses likes to have fun with their hair. It's great for our business. Look at Sienna Miller now. When her hair was long, she was still beautiful but she looked like everyone else. Now you can really see her. She has her own look, and a real identity. You can do so many more things with a shorter haircut. You can change it artistically, roll it or straighten it or wear it high. Sometimes, you need to push your limits. If they get a push from their stylists, [women] might be more willing to accept the change. Men are more aware of what's happening now than ever before. They are not stuck in one traditional way of looking at women. That is one of the reasons women are more daring. You don't have to look the same, with long boring hair, to be attractive and modern. If a woman is really attached to long hair she can do some crazy things to it, because she wants a change and doesn't want to cut it. Sometimes a stylist needs to tell a woman that she needs a cut instead of a crazy color or perm for a change. They end up damaging their hair and not being happy with it." Fabrice Gili

LIMP LOCKS

The Buzz from the Beauty Editor

When I was in college, I was hanging out with a girlfriend when we decided to do each other's hair. Her hair was superfine and silky-smooth, and as I tried to put it up in a French twist, it slipped out of my grasp and fell down around her shoulders. It was so slippery, it was nearly impossible to style. It was so different than my own thick, curly hair, and I was fascinated. I have always thought girls with fine hair had it easy, because their hair never gets big, bushy, or out of control, but trying to style her hair that day, I realized that every hair type has its challenges.

Insider Information from the Beauty Bunch

Good Order

"If you have extremely fine hair, apply the conditioner first and then shampoo. You will still get all of the benefits from the conditioner, and the shampoo will remove any residue that could weigh down your hair." Nathaniel Hawkins

Blow-Dry Boost

"My big tip for every single person, because we all want some volume, is to dry the roots up and out, so that they have volume, rather than drying them down. Part hair to the right and blow it up and out, and then flip it over and do the same thing on the other side. You don't want a flat head." Jessica Tingley

Limp Locks

"Fine, limp hair can't be layered to death. Add some weight by cutting it more bluntly, and using thickening products to give it bulk. This will give volume to the hair. Your hairdresser should be able to tell you what thickening or volumizing products to use." Michael O'Rourke

Pump Up the Volume

"If you have fine, limp hair and you'd like more volume, wait half an hour after washing your hair to start styling. The heat from the hair-dryer can actually blast your hair flat, so that there is no volume. And if you apply hair products on wet hair, the products will mix with the water to weigh the hair down. Let it air-dry, and comb through it with fingers to let the air circulate for half an hour first." Damien Miano

Fine Print

"Really fine, limp hair has two options: it can be worn really short with lots of layers to give it body, or it can be worn in a blunt bob, all one length. If you wear it longer with layers, it will empty out the texture and be overlayered, and that will accentuate the thinness of it. Short is really the best option for fine hair." Fabrice Gili

Fine Products

"For fine hair, try a volumizing shampoo. The technology in these shampoos fattens the hair. It's the same technology they use in lip plumpers." Jessica Tingley

Short Answer

"The best cut and style for very fine, limp hair is one which accents the client's face, not her hair. That said, shorter is better with this type of hair, but how short and what style is going to depend on the individual." Peter Lamas

PRODUCT PRINCIPLES

The Buzz from the Beauty Editor

My bathroom is filled with so many hair products, it looks like a salon. I've got five different types of conditioner, three shampoos, and countless styling products. The pros agree that there are some products worth splurging on, and others where you could stand to save. They just don't agree on what those products are. Here, their suggestions for buying hair products, whatever your budget.

Insider Information from the Beauty Bunch

Kudos for Kerastase

Several members of the Beauty Bunch are fans of the French hair-care line, even those with lines of their own, like Ric Pipino and Charles Worthington. Worthington added the Best Hair Treatment category just so he could nominate Kerastase Masquintense, which is also the choice of Pipino, Danielle Browning, and Fabien Roussel. Roussel swears by the Masquintense for Fine Hair for its ability to make hair smooth and silky, and offers these instructions: "Apply onto half-inch sections of hair, and massage treatment into sections. Then wrap in a hot towel and let process for ten minutes. Emulsify with warm water and rinse thoroughly with cool water." Shauna Raisch and Jan Marini both count on Kerastase Oleo-Relax Serum to get curly hair smooth and sleek, and Marini offers this tip: "Put it on your hair when it's wet, and then style as usual. It looks like an oil but it won't weigh hair down. It disappears and makes your hair as smooth as silk and able to resist humidity. And it leaves hair in great condition." Kattia Solano offers a complete Kerastase prescription for a smoother blow-out on medium to thick hair: Nutritive Bain Satin 2 Shampoo, Resistance Age Recharge Masque (as a conditioner), and Nutritive Lait Nutri-Sculpt for styling. "It smoothes out the frizz for the blow-dry," she says. And when asked whether it's possible to shield hair from the sun, Shauna Raisch said emphatically, "The answer is a big yes! Sun-protection products are the answer. Kerastase Soleil products are made for the sun. [There's a] shampoo, conditioner, two types of sunscreen for the hair, a detangler/protectant, and the niftiest thing of all, a gel product to block out chlorine and salt water. Sun care—don't leave home without it!" But not all of the pros unequivocally applauded Kerastase. Rachel Lindy likes the styling products for a quick fix, but feels that the shampoos and conditioners contain too much alcohol, making them drying when used regularly.

Overnight Success

"Frédéric Fekkai Overnight Hair Repair has a new technology that really gets into the cortex. It's an overnight mask that's like skin care for the hair." Jessica Tingley

Splurge Suggestions

"Shampoo and conditioner are the most important items, so spend your money here because cheap shampoos and conditioners have so many perfumes and waxes. They build up in the hair and make it oilier. Also, with cheap products, the scent stays in the hair and hair won't look as shiny or healthy. Then you need a clarifier, which strips the hair, and it's a constant cycle." Rachel Lindy

Spend to Save

"Cheap products, cheap hair. If you use products that are inexpensive, because they're filled with cheap chemicals, your hair will reflect that. Additionally, you'll find that cheaper products are not very concentrated, so you go through them quickly. In the long run, you're probably not saving any money. I recommend buying from a salon or beauty-supply store, not the drugstore." Peter Lamas

Defeating Dryness

"The most common complaint is that the hair doesn't grow as fast as it's supposed to, and that it's dry. In the summertime, everyone wants longer hair. Use a hair mask, like Kerastase, once a week for half an hour. Before going to the beach, put a mask on to protect the hair, and rinse it out after coming home." David Cotteblanche

Style Splurge

"It's good to spend on shampoo and conditioner, but most importantly, get good styling products to make your life easier. They make your life so much simpler. Spend the money on products that help control your hair or give you volume quickly and easily." Michael O'Rourke

Splurge on Style

"[I recommend] splurging on styling products when you find a product that works. The most inexpensive gel we sell here is what works on my hair, but if it cost one hundred dollars, I'd spend it because it works on my hair. I was lucky because it's a cheap one. Generally speaking, more expensive products perform better. Find a product that you like, and if you like the way it feels, looks, and works, nothing shy of that is going to look as good. But you need to change it periodically. You could not spend as much on shampoo, but find a standard shampoo that doesn't strip your hair." Damien Miano

Spendthrift

"Splurge on a great haircut, a good blow-dryer, and a good shampoo. Shampoo is really important. It can strip hair and make it frizzy or make it heavy and limp and greasy. A great shampoo gets you started on the right foot, and then you don't need ten products to make it look good. And if you have a bad haircut, there is nothing you can do with it. You end up spending half an hour in the morning to make it look decent, which is ridiculous." Jessica Tingley

Save on Style

"You can get away with spending less on shine serums. Frizz Ease, for example, is not as expensive as the Kerastase serum. And gels and mousses are all basically the same. They have a high alcohol content. That's what makes them work, and less product is better than more product, unless you have curly hair." Rachel Lindy

City Solutions

"Hair is your ultimate bespoke fashion accessory because you wear it every day. Especially in cities, your hair needs special attention to counteract the effects of climate and the elements." Charles Worthington

Star Endorsement

"Eva Longoria uses Big Sexy Hair Spray & Play Hairspray, and travels with it. She recommends us all over, [which is] very nice." Michael O'Rourke

Care First

"The most important thing [to splurge on] is shampoo and conditioner. Use a good hair mask. It's very important for the hair, like the skin. That's the best thing you can do. A lot of people spend a lot and use a lot of styling products, and it's better not to use too much mousse or anything. You don't have to use as much as you think." David Cotteblanche

TOOLS AND TECHNIQUES

The Buzz from the Beauty Editor

I don't consider myself a gadget geek, but I'm fascinated by the tools used by professional hairstylists. The right combs, brushes, blow-dryers, and flatirons open up a world of possibilities; they have the ability to literally transform your hair.

Insider Information from the Beauty Bunch

Ions Explained

"The most important thing to know is that hair has a negative charge anyway, and pollutants are positive and are attracted to that negative charge. Ionic products stimulate the negative charge, so that hair can protect itself against pollutants. Nanotechnology is a silver derivative, and it's nature's way of boosting the hair's negative charge." Michael O'Rourke

A Better Brush

"The Spornette G-78 is the best styling brush. It has been featured on *In Style*'s Best list. Pierre Michel and Constance Hartnett at Frédéric Fekkai recommend it for blow-outs." Jimmy Vanegas

High and Dry

"Invest in an ionic dryer—it's even more important than the shampoo! A good ionic dryer or ceramic iron—the kinds that the pros use—is hotter, which makes the hair shiny and dries it faster. I recommend the T3 Tourmaline Ionic Hair Dryer." Rachel Lindy

Ponytail Primer

"Never use a ponytail band that has a metal clasp. The tension of the metal on the hair creates breakage." Nathaniel Hawkins

Party Prep

"If you're going out after work and don't feel like washing your hair, try Velcro rollers," advises Barry Reitman. "Take sections of hair the width of the roller and, starting from the middle front, roll it back. Take another roller and do the section behind that, and so on. You'll probably have three rollers down the middle and one on either side. Add a light mist of hair spray, and ten minutes later, remove the Velcro rollers. Don't brush your hair. Just flip your head upside down and run your fingers through your hair. It's a very glamorous look, it only takes ten minutes, and it's done on dry hair." Nathaniel Hawkins agrees. "Velcro rollers are magic. Wrap them in your hair and spray lightly with an aerosol hair spray. Add some heat and then let cool for twenty minutes. It is one of the easiest ways to create shiny hair that's full of body, and it will totally transform your hair."

Finger Cues

"The most indispensable tool for hair styling is your fingers. I don't like styles which are heavily dependent on brushes, combs, curlers, or blow-dryers." Peter Lamas

Isn't It Ionic

"I like ionic treatments. Like any chemical process, it works best on natural hair. But if your hair is too dry, it's too much. After a certain point, it doesn't work the way it's supposed to. Ionic blow-dryers are excellent. The best ionic products work on slightly dry hair." David Cotteblanche

Ionic Hot Air

"I think some [ionic products] are just gimmicks, to be honest. I have clients who use them and those who don't, and I'm not sure there's a difference. I don't know about these negative and positive charges. Hair is dead matter. I don't believe there's a dryer that spews out miraculous air." Damien Miano

Top Tool

"I love the T3 Tourmaline 1-Inch Ceramic Hair Straightener. You can use it to flatiron, to turn up the ends, and you can wrap the hair around it and slowly slide it down the hair to get the most romantic loose curl you've ever seen. It's two tools in one: it straightens and curls. For blow-dryers, the Barbar Italy 5000 is light and dependable, and the Solano is the standard that most hairstylists use." Barry Reitman

Best Brushes

"Invest in an excellent brush and comb. Mason Pearson brushes are exquisite because they last many years. Their bristles last, the pneumatic cushion doesn't break, and because of the little hole in the frame, water drains after washing the brush and mold doesn't build up underneath the cushion. Brushing cleans and massages the scalp, so brush your hair as often as possible. The cleansing, refreshing, and stimulating effect will carry you and your hair throughout the day. Brush your hair while leaning forward and then while you are standing upright. Roll the brush into the hairline. Go from one ear to the other. Long, deep strokes will increase blood circulation to the scalp. Comb or brush your hair when it is about two-thirds dry. This avoids loss of elasticity. If you don't like the visual effect brushing has on your hair, brush before going to bed. If your hair is very curly and you really can't get a brush through it, replace brushing with finger massage." Linda Deslauriers

Simply Indispensable

"The best [most indispensable] tool is the blow-dryer. You can use it to diffuse, with fingers, with a brush. It's very versatile." David Cotteblanche

Brush with Greatness

"If you are struggling with your brushes," says Damien Miano, "you should invest in good ones. Cheap brushes don't create the right movement. Splurge on a good brush, good styling tools, and good styling products. I love the Mason Pearson mixed-bristle brushes; the ones that are all-natural don't go through the hair as well. They don't get to the scalp. The mixed-bristle brushes work better when you style the hair, because they have a little more pull, which is great for styling and stimulating." Ric Pipino is also a fan of Mason Pearson brushes, voting them the best for blow-outs.

Comb and Collected

"Wooden combs feel great. Make sure they don't have splinters. You can oil them with olive oil to make them smooth. Antistatic combs made of rubber instead of plastic reduce the fireworks on your head." Linda Deslauriers

THE BIG BLOW-OUT

The Buzz from the Beauty Editor

When I find myself in a dry climate, I have my hair blown out, just for a change. Straight hair is sleek, sophisticated, and polished, and a nice change from my usual curls. I am also convinced that curly hair brings out my sweet, bubbly side, but when my hair is straight, I can have a little bit more attitude.

Insider Information from the Beauty Bunch

Blow-Out Basics

"There are a few things you definitely need for a good blow-out. Number one, you need your product, some kind of a smoothing serum. Apply just a nickel- to a quarter-size amount, depending on how much hair you have and how curly or frizzy it is, on clean, damp hair. I like Sudzz FX Zenyth Frizz Eliminator. It makes hair really shiny and smooth, and it smells great. You also need a professional blow-dryer. Technique is not the only reason that a stylist is able to get your hair so shiny and smooth. It's also the heat. Heat makes the cuticle lie down smooth and makes hair shiny. The new trend is the ionic ceramic dryer, and these are the best. What a difference! The T3 Tourmaline Ionic Dryer is much lighter than the old kind: half a pound to one pound as opposed to the five-pound weight of a standard dryer. And it dries the hair twice as fast. The only downside is that they are very fragile. Finally, you need a great brush. I get bored and get new brushes every couple of months, but right now my favorite is the T3 Tourmaline Ionic Ceramic Brush. A good product, a good round brush, and a good blow-dryer are the three most important things you need. And clips to section your hair off. It helps so much to get the rest of the hair out of your way. Once you have what you need, it's just about practicing. As for straightening irons, I don't need to use them because I can get hair really straight. The problem with straightening irons is that people are uneducated about them and fry their hair. Your hair has to be one hundred percent bone dry before you use it. There should be no moisture. If you get that steam effect, you're fizzling your hair. Once your hair is completely dry, go over each section once or twice, no more. Going over the same piece over and over again damages the hair, and so does holding it on the hair, and it won't get it any smoother." Rachel Lindy

Beat the Heat

"I always apply any type of silicone product to the hair before applying heat. Heat causes the silicone to fuse to the hair, creating a beautiful supernatural shine while smoothing the hair shaft." Nathaniel Hawkins

High and Dry

"Start blow-drying the front of your hair first. That's what's framing your face. If you start at the back, by the time you get to the front you are tired or late. And then flip your head upside down and dry it from underneath. It's much quicker." Barry Reitman

Ionic Setback

"Ionic blow-dryers work almost too well. They make hair too shiny, too slippery, and too flat. It won't hold a curl, even with the ionic curlers. Heat makes your hair hold a shape, but with an ionic dryer, it won't hold any shape." Jessica Tingley

Top Technique

"Don't use any tools at first. Turn your head upside down and blow-dry upside down. Dry it completely first, unless it's very curly. Apply product with a comb, when you use a mousse, and do it section by section. Don't do it all with your hands. Using a comb will make it more even." David Cotteblanche

Blow-Dry Boosters

"Try a leave-in conditioner and a 'defrisant' before you blow-dry. Sudzz FX is only twenty dollars for a huge bottle that can last you a year. It's a great middle-of-the-road-priced product that keeps hair from getting frizzy, adds shine, and holds your blow-out." Rachel Lindy

Blow-Dry Boundaries

"Turn off your blow-dryer before your hair is dry. This way you will not overdry it. If you must use a blow-dryer on a daily basis, protect yourself with a Q-Link to minimize electromagnetic pollution. One study showed that male hairdressers have the highest occurrence of breast cancer among male professionals." Linda Deslauriers

Blow-Dry Buzz

To recreate a salon blow-out at home, "you must have the right products! The best thing is to just spring for the salon 'do. If you have curly hair that has been blown straight, stay out of the humidity! Use Kerastase Oleo-Relax Serum and Fixative to lock out humidity." Shauna Raisch

Towel Technique

"Save on blow-drying time by towel-drying your hair first. Take one, two, or even three towels and press out the excess water; leave the last towel on your head as a turban. If your hair is longer than two inches, don't rub your hair with a towel after washing. Instead, press gently onto your hair. This way you avoid entanglement, breakage, and loss of elasticity." Linda Deslauriers

THE BATTLE OF THE BULGE:
HANDLING CURLY, THICK, OR FRIZZY HAIR

The Buzz from the Beauty Editor
Curly-haired women, like myself, have a sort of silent sorority. We analyze each other's curls, stalk each other's stylists, and stop each other on the streets to get the product scoop. Once, at a dinner out with my husband, I was so obsessed by another woman's beautiful curls that I literally couldn't stop staring at her through the entire meal. With that kind of obsession, we want all the tips we can get. Fortunately, this chapter features scores of them.

Insider Information from the Beauty Bunch

Frizz Fighting

"Frizzy hair can happen everywhere. Some people can get it under control with specific products, like glosses, creams, or straightening balms. If it's crazy-frizzy, and hard to control, the best way to tame it is with a blow-dryer and a flatiron. If someone has good curly hair, then they can work with it, but many people don't know how to work with hair that's frizzy. It won't curl properly, and it's not as neat as they would like it do be, so they blow it out." Jessica Tingley

Fight Frizz

"You have to use extra product on [hair to fight frizz]. It's difficult when it's really raining. There's not much you can do. Put on some extra finishing product. Using olive oil is very good, or anything that will pull down your hair." David Cotteblanche

Thick Is Beautiful
"Women with thick hair have to stop saying that their hair is awful. Their hair is the best. That's the gift of life if you can get hair like that. Just use bigger brushes. The most beautiful people with the most beautiful hair have the most complaints." Michael O'Rourke

Carving and Slicing
"Straight hair is about thinking in the box, but curly hair is all about thinking out of the box. It's important to listen to the curl. What we do with carving and slicing is we create a seat underneath the curl so that the upper curl fits into that piece like a puzzle and lies nicely. The curls are cut so that they fit together; you don't get that pyramid effect." Ouidad

Long Layers
"The best cut and style for curly hair is long, layered pieces." Peter Lamas

Beautiful Extremes
"There are two ways to approach curly hair. You can get rid of the bulk with a pretty short cut with a lot of layers, or let in the curls in an all natural way and leave the length. Anything in between is kind of a problem because it shrinks a lot and has too much volume, and that's not too flattering. So you need to either get rid of most of the curls or keep most of them." Fabrice Gili

Short End
"This has happened very few times, but we have actually sent a few clients away without cutting their hair because the hair is too short. If curly hair is too short, there isn't the length that's needed to form the curl pattern. We tell them to come back in a couple of months, when their hair has grown out, and they can't believe it. But you have to be honest and understand how to work with hair and balance it out. When you cut a client's hair, you enter into a contract with them. You have to honor that contract." Ouidad

Curl Cut
"I don't think there is one style [for curly hair]. It's better with very curly hair to leave it longer. It's extremes. It can be cut short or long. In between, it's very hard to manage." David Cotteblanche

Redirecting the Curl
"No one is really happy with very tight curls, or frizz. For women who are fighting their natural curls, one way of dealing with it is to redirect the curl with a perm to soften it a bit. A perm can help you redirect the natural wave to make it easier to take care of, and using bigger rollers can make hair much smoother and more modern, and will also get rid of frizz. Big rollers will create loose curls and smaller rollers will create tight curls. For very coarse, curly hair, it's better to have a soft, redirected curl than straight hair. Don't fight nature. Just work on making your natural curl easier. Curly hair is very pretty, but you might just need to find a way to make it more manageable." Fabrice Gili

Mane Mistake
"The biggest mistake curly-haired women make is having their hair thinned or layered. You cannot thin hair out randomly or texturize it. You have to think about the regrowth. The curls have to be strategically cut and designed to fit into each other or the hair will grow out wild and frizzy." Ouidad

Reigning in Ringlets
"Curly hair is its own kind. It has a completely different process to anything else. Most curly hair has

got volume to it. If you don't know how to handle it, it can be unmanageable. For every half an inch, cut hair lightly at the root. Remove twenty-five percent of hair lower to the root, and then you'll have space in between the hair and the curl falls into that negative space, whereas before it stacked up on itself and became enormous. Cut the space in between so that the curl falls into itself, and that way it moves beautifully. You have to handle it differently, but it's the most magnificent hair. I love it." Michael O'Rourke

Move Over Mullet

"One big, big, big mistake that curly-haired women make is having the top part of their hair cut short for height and volume. For straight hair, cutting it short does give it volume, but that doesn't work for curly hair. There isn't enough length to form the curl and it ends up flat, and looks like a mullet." Ouidad

Curl Talk

"I cut curly hair like I cut straight hair. I just expect it to shrink up. It has to look good, whether you style it straight or curly. I never want to thin out or razor-cut curly hair, because it makes it frizzier and twice as big. Leave a little conditioner in it when you get out of the shower, and try not to touch it when it's drying. Don't scrunch. You will just separate the curls and they won't form. After it's dry, shake it up and shape it. In California, the climate is so dry that women have to encourage their curls, whereas people in humid climates like Florida love curls, because they work so well there." Jessica Tingley

Straight Talk about Straighteners

"Perms and straighteners are actually the same product, the same chemical; it's just the way that they are used, with either a flatiron or rollers, that is different. A perm or a straightener is essential if you want to totally change the shape of your hair, but if it's too strong you will overdry the hair and ruin it. That's why a lot of those Japanese straightening treatments lead to breakage. At one point, the hair is not going to react properly. A straightener can change the quality of the hair drastically because it changes the cuticle of the hair and it's hard to come back. Even coloring your hair for many years will cause it to straighten eventually. It changes the shape of the hair so that it's not as shiny or flexible. Over time, the chemicals change the hair. So go really, really slow; try not to make drastic changes in color or texture. Beauty should enhance a woman naturally, instead of being extreme. It's like a brunette who goes blonde right away and it doesn't go with her coloring. I think it's all about trends. In the last two or three years, the trend was all about straight hair, worn long with long bangs, and now the trend is coming back with everything more loose and rock-and-roll and not too 'done' looking. If you have a permanent-straightening treatment and your hair is pin-straight, you can't do anything with it. You wake up with the hair looking exactly the same every morning, and you're stuck with it. The modern woman wants to change her hair two or three times a day. You don't want to leave the client stuck in one style all the time. I push them to play with their natural hair and I think that's where the fun is." Fabrice Gili

Avoiding your Zzzz's

"A very tight, z-shaped curl pattern is a sign of dehydration. Use a conditioning treatment." Ouidad

Curl Saver

To save time when styling curly hair, "put product in your hair and, in the car, use your fingers to shape the curls." Michael O'Rourke

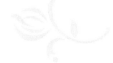

Decoding Your Curls

"With the average curly head of hair, it's normal to have three or four different types of curl. Some areas will be tighter than others, or frizzier. Visually, you should be able to determine the type of curls that you have. As far as texture, the majority of curly hair is baby-fine. This is one case where looks are deceiving. It looks big and tough, but it isn't. I've seen a mixture of fine curly hair and coarse curly hair on one head. You can determine your hair's texture by touch, and by looking at an individual strand of hair. You'll be able to see if it's fine or coarse. But don't look at the actual curl to determine that; straighten it out and look." Ouidad

Curly Top Tip

"Use Phytotherathrie Phytocurl Shampoo and Phytosesame Conditioner. Wrap hair around finger and let dry into beautiful locks." Fabien Roussel

Top Tools

"Your tools are your fingers with curly hair. And a wide-toothed comb for detangling in the shower, so that there's less frizz." Ouidad

Picking Products

"When I started out, there were no products for curly hair. Today, there are so many and they still don't get it. Curly-hair products need to be water-soluble and light; you cannot use heavy products on curly hair even though your psyche might tell you to weigh it down and control it. I have always had to talk women out of the heavy stuff and into the light stuff. It's very important that you understand that you don't need to weigh it down. So look for products that are light and water-soluble." Ouidad

Curl Control

"The biggest mistake with curly hair is to cut it in a medium length. It should be either short or long, preferably long. Medium lengths make hair look like it's a ball. It won't have a good shape. Curly hair in a medium length is not very flattering. Leave length through the top and through the front. Nothing is worse than curly hair with short bangs. The problem is more the length than the specific style, because it comes down to how you handle it, how you style it. Overlayered is really a mistake. You want long layers." Damien Miano

Curly Tactics

"To style frizzy, curly hair, apply a light gel or cream and let air-dry. With a large curling iron, take random sections and wrap hair around the iron. Hold for a few seconds, then release and pull down curl. This will give beautiful, sexy curls." Kattia Solano

Peak Condition

"If your hair is in a corkscrew shape, the outer layer is not protected, so you need a deep treatment every two weeks. If your hair is healthy and conditioned internally—by using an intensive conditioner like the Ouidad Deep Treatment—it will have its own internal weight, and you won't need to weigh it down with heavy products. Using silicone or wax products will repel moisture and dehydrate your hair even more. If your hair is filled properly, at the molecular level, you don't have to worry about humidity." Ouidad

Wondrous Waves

"Towel-dry hair, then apply product for texture. I recommend Kerastase Nutritive Crème Nutri-Sculpt. Create two 'Princess Leia' buns. Blow-dry or let dry naturally. Loosen buns and then you will have sexy waves." Kattia Solano

Curl Control

"Curly hair is hard because it is such a personal thing; a lot depends on your specific curly hair. Everyone's curls are different. The most important thing starting out is the haircut. If you have no curl on top, just on the bottom, you're going to have that pyramid-head effect. You need to balance it out all over with long soft layers, and long layers around the face. As for products, you have to experiment and mix a lot of different things together. Everyone seems to have their own little concoction. Use a leave-in conditioner and start scrunching it in the hair—even though I hate that word because its so eighties. Sometimes I will put the product in and twist big sections around my finger and just leave them to create bigger, looser curls. There's a line called CurlFriends that works great, although I don't like the scent or the packaging. I recommend their Replenish Leave-In Conditioner and the Rejuvenate Texturizing Mist. Besides a leave-in conditioner, you'll also want another product, but it's hard to say which one, because it's so individual. Kerastase Elasto-Curl Weightless Mousse works well on fine, curly hair, but thick, coarse hair needs something more emollient, like the Elasto-Curl Definition Forming Cream. You don't want a gel because you don't want your hair to feel hard. Don't brush your hair when you come out of the shower; just finger-comb it. If you let it dry naturally, it turns out better than with a diffuser. You'll have more frizz and more body with a diffuser. If you choose to use a diffuser, there is a diffuser attachment for the T3 Tourmaline Ionic Dryer." Rachel Lindy

CITY SECRETS

After opening his first American salon in SoHo, British superstylist Charles Worthington commissioned a study to learn about the hair habits of American women. This is what he discovered:

35 percent of American women would rather have great hair for life than great sex for life

79 percent of American women spend up to twenty minutes every morning styling their hair, with 70 percent of women washing their hair in the morning

43 percent of women cite time spent on styling as the main factor in determining how good their hair looks

Bad hair days result in dramatic reactions, including fighting with boyfriend/husband (22 percent), wearing distracting fashion accessories (21 percent), and even refusing to leave the house (18 percent)

The biggest hair complaint is damage and dryness (38 percent) followed by frizz (31 percent)

The ultimate hair wish is to have more volume and bounce (35 percent), followed by an equal 25 percent wishing for locks that are not damaged by the elements (sun, wind, water) and are frizz-free

Curls rule as the top summer-night styling trend, being most popular in Tampa (36 percent), Phoenix (33 percent), and Chicago (30 percent), while straight and sleek is the New York trend

Cameron Diaz has the favored summer hairstyle according to 45 percent of women

Women in Phoenix have the cleanest hair in America with 63 percent washing their hair daily, yet they also suffer the most from damage and dryness

44 percent of Phoenix women blame climate for making hair dry and staticky and to that end, 42 percent wear their hair up in ponytails, barrettes, or braids during the summer (the highest across the cities queried)

Phoenix women prefer curls, with a sizable 42 percent using curling irons at home

Hairspray is the top styler of choice for 40 percent of Phoenix and Tampa women

29 percent of women in Phoenix have fought with their boyfriend or husband because of a bad hair day

Phoenix women favor Drew Barrymore's free-spirited locks

Women in San Francisco earned the title Best Hair in America by having the fewest bad hair days

San Francisco women also tend to be the most relaxed and minimalist about their hair, and generally prefer a no-fuss straight look with minimal styling time and tools

Bay City women tend to wear their hair straight at all times—weekdays, weekends, nights out. They spend the least time styling their hair, with 50 percent zipping through styling in less than ten minutes whereas nearly a quarter of women in Chicago spend up to thirty minutes styling their locks

72 percent describe their look as low-maintenance and natural, with 41 percent not using any hair styling tools and 75 percent saying they do not have bad hair days

Lucy Liu's straight style earned top reviews in San Francisco

New York women are the most frizzed-out and favor a naturally wavy look during the day and a sleek, straight style at night. They reported frizz as their main hair problem (40 percent) with weather most affecting how they style their tresses

During summer days, New Yorkers (61 percent of whom describe their look as "downtown") prefer to wear their hair naturally wavy or curly (more so than counterparts in Phoenix) and then straighten it when going out at night

New York City women are the most frequent night-shampooers (38 percent)

When having a bad hair day, New York City women are slightly dramatic, with 15 percent admitting to canceling a date and 5 percent admitting to calling in sick to work

Tampa ladies complain of damage, dryness (43 percent), and limp locks (33 percent) attributed to a sunny, humid climate

Women in Tampa are the most dramatic when having a bad hair day, with 30 percent fighting with a boyfriend or husband and 24 percent refusing to leave the house

Tampa ladies are most likely to rely on the expertise of hairstylists (57 percent), followed by San Francisco women (55 percent)

Fans of curling their locks when going out at night, Tampa women mainly use two hair styling products, with hairspray being the most popular (40 percent)

Chicago women recognize the importance of good hair, investing more time in styling, straightening, and experimenting with their locks

Windy City women are most swayed by a lifetime of great hair over great sex, according to 39 percent of respondents

Similar to New York women, 71 percent of Chicago ladies are experimental with hair looks when going out at night and invest more time on their hair

Nearly a quarter of Chicago respondents devote up to thirty minutes styling their locks

More than 1 in 5 Chicago women play it straight at home, more than counterparts in other cities

During summer days, 40 percent of women in the Windy City wear their hair up in ponytails, barrettes, and braids

25 percent of Chicago women complained of limp locks and are the most frequent mousse users (17 percent)

Survey courtesy of Charles Worthington

THE PRODUCT FILES

Shampoos

The Buzz from the Beauty Editor

Effective two-in-one shampoo/conditioner products are an urban myth; they neither clean nor condition very well. My ideal shampoo is one that cleanses effectively without stripping. I never want my hair to feel squeaky. All shampoos clean, but since they're rinsed out so quickly, few leave your hair with lasting benefits. If you have long hair, concentrate shampoo at the roots and on the scalp, rather than on the ends. I pour some shampoo into my palm, spread it around between my hands, and then apply it to the roots only. The length of my hair gets a sufficient dose of shampoo when I rinse. More than that, and dry ends ensue. My favorites are Komenuka-Bijin Hair Shampoo, $33, and Charles Worthington Dream Hair Heavenly Hairwash Outrageously Rich Shampoo, $6.

What the Pros Choose

The only similarity between the shampoo preferences of the pros is that they pick unique, even obscure products. No Pantene for these professionals. Pros who stood by their own, often eponymous lines included Oribe (Oribe Protein Infusion), Ric Pipino (Pipino Wash Away Purifying Gentle Shampoo), Peter Thomas Roth (Peter Thomas Roth Botanical Oasis Shampoo), June Jacobs (June Jacobs Citrus Shampoo), and Charles Worthington (Charles Worthington Results Moisture Seal Glossing Shampoo). Seaworthy products include Jim Miller's California North Sea-Blast Shampoo (which holds color and prevents "pool hair") and Dee DeLuca-Mattos' Ecru New York Sea Clean Shampoo. Shampoos designed to produce specific results include Bumble and bumble Thickening (Wende Zomnir); Pureology Hydrate (Meredith Green); and The Vital Image Renewal (Linda Deslauriers). Rachel Lindy raves about Sudzz FX, "Their shampoos have no sulfates. The entire line is terrific and smells amazing." Two Phytotherathrie shampoos make the cut: Phytolactum (Anthony Rocanello) and Phytonectar (Fabien Roussel). Other picks include Robert Kree Clean Daily Moisturizing Shampoo (Mala Elhassan), Fresh Soda Shampoo (Hara Glick), Redken (Galit Strugano), Deesse's (Nelson Chan), Komenuka-Bijin Shampoo (Meg Thompson), and Frédéric Fekkai (another pick from June Jacobs). Barry Reitman swears by Schwartzkopf and Paul Brown shampoos for color-treated hair, and is also a fan of Paul Mitchell shampoos. Darin Birchler loves any of the Kerastase Nutritive shampoos (which include Bain Satin 1, 2, and 3; Bain Oleo-Relax; and Bain Elasto-Curl) for their ability to leave hair silky and smooth, while Ric Pipino recommends Kerastase Nutritive Bain Satin 2 for dry hair and Shauna Raisch loves Kerastase Bain Apres-Soleil. Shan Albert swears by Sircuit Liquid Crystal Hydrating Hair Bath because it's free of harmful ingredients, produces loads of luxurious lather, and allows her to comb her color-treated hair sans conditioner.

Conditioners

The Buzz from the Beauty Editor

I go through three bottles of conditioner for every one bottle of shampoo. My long, thick, dry hair demands loads of it, and soaks it right up. That's why, even though I sometimes buy shampoo and conditioner in pairs from the same line, they rarely stay that way. Usually, you'll find my shower crammed with a mess of mismatched products. If your hair is long, thick, and dry enough to handle it, use your regular conditioner as a leave-in. Simply skip the rinse, comb it through to detangle, and style as usual. Your conditioner will serve as your base styling product, and you'll need to use less of your other styling products. My thick, curly hair would be out of control if I rinsed out my conditioner; it's the only thing that really seems to keep it in check. I use all of the conditioners on my list as leave-ins, and they do a great job of keeping my curls coiled and controlled. My favorites are Pantene Pro-V Hydrating Curls Conditioner, $5, Ouidad Curl Quencher Conditioner, $12, and John Frieda Frizz-Ease Smooth Control Defrizzing & Nourishing Conditioner/Extra Strength Formula, $5.

What the Pros Choose

Again, the pros go for the exclusive and eclectic. Conditioners mentioned by more than one pro include Bumble and bumble (Julie Hewett and Wende Zomnir, who specifies the Thickening Conditioner), Kerastase (Hewett's second pick, and the choice of Fabien Roussel, who swears by Masquintense, Shauna Raisch, who loves Lait Vital Protein Conditioning Milk, and Oribe, who chose Crème Richesse), and Crede Treatment (Nelson Chan and Rachel Lindy). Lindy loves Crede because "it's very silkening. If you highlight your hair and blow it out, use a mask at least once a week. This is a great hair mask. People with dry hair can use it every day."

Roussel also has another pick, ISH Ionic Conditioning Treatment. Anthony Rocanello is a Phytotherathrie fan, and his pick for top conditioner is Phytokarite. Barry Reitman raves about J. Beverly Hills Masque Conditioner, which he calls a "magic bullet for curly hair. It has a great minty smell and works on hair that is dry, curly, or color-treated. You can leave it on or rinse it out, and it's absolutely incredible." Eponymous picks include Pipino Pure Happiness Daily Replenishing Conditioner (Pipino says that it won't weigh hair down with daily use), Peter Thomas Roth Botanical Oasis Conditioner, and Charles Worthington Results Superconditioner. Other picks include Robert Kree Moist Moisturizing Finishing Rinse (Mala Elhassan), Terax Crema (Darin Birchler, who loves how it leaves dry, thick, over-processed hair soft and pliable), The Vital Image Hair Therapy (Linda Deslauriers), Komenuka-Bijin Hair Treatment (Meg Thompson), Rene Furterer Fioravanti Silkening Conditioner (Oribe), California North Watermint Conditioner (Jim Miller), Modern Organic Products Daily Rinse Conditioner (Hara Glick), Redken Extreme Conditioner (Galit Strugano), Ecru New York Luxe Treatment Shampoo (chosen in place of conditioner by Dee DeLuca-Mattos), Pureology Hydrate Condition (Meredith Green), and Sircuit Crystal Crème Revitalizing Hair Conditioner (Shan Albert).

Styling Products

The Buzz from the Beauty Editor
I have never met anyone with thicker hair than my own, so I am the ultimate tester for products designed for those with thick or curly hair. I always apply conditioner towards the beginning of my shower, leave it in for the duration, and then detangle my hair at the end. Invariably, I shed enough hair to make a hairpiece, and, invariably, it ends up on the walls of my shower. (Sticking hair to

the shower is the quickest way to get it off your hands, I've found.) Unfortunately, since my husband has baby-fine blonde hair, there's no mistaking that the wads of dark hair in the shower are mine. He's nicknamed them "shower creatures." Looking for a quick, inexpensive way to make medium-to-very curly hair beautiful and bouncy? After shampooing, apply your regular conditioner and leave it in while you shave, scrub, etc. Then, before stepping out of the shower, use a wide-toothed comb to detangle your hair. Do not rinse your conditioner out. (Even if it's not a leave-in. Trust me. It works.) Immediately post-shower (while hair is still dripping wet), apply enough Aussie 3 Minute Miracle or Queen Helene Cholesterol to coat the surface of the hair, going easy on the top of your head. (Too much product at the roots and at the hairline will look white and can flake off.) Then, apply a light coat of gel, serum, or your other favorite shine and hold enhancing products to the length of your hair. Once you get the hang of it, it's practically foolproof. My other favorite products include Redken Solid Water 06 Wet Set Gel, $14.95, and FX Curl Booster Fixative Gel, $6.

What the Pros Choose

Redken gets two votes in this category (Hara Glick chose Sharp Edge Whipped Graphic Spray Wax and Nelson Chan picked Outshine Anti-Frizz Polishing Milk), while Kerastase receives three nods: Julie Hewett; Anthony Rocanello, who specifies the Lumi-Extract; and Shauna Raisch, who loves the Crème Nutri-Sculpt. Gel lovers include Wende Zomnir (Phytotherathrie Pro Sculpting Gel) and Mala Elhassan (Graham Webb Nolita Grit Gel), while spray fans

include Barry Reitman (MOP Lemongrass Lift), Dee DeLuca-Mattos (Ecru New York Sunlight Holding), Charles Worthington (Charles Worthington Results Make Over Blow Dry), and Linda Deslauriers (Anthony Morrocco Five Elements Diamond Crystal Mist Conditioner and Moisturizer). Other picks include Hamadi Shea styling products (Meg Thompson), Bumble and bumble (Hewett's second pick), L'Oreal Professionel Liss Extreme Smoothing Cream (Gabrielle Ophals), Phytotherathrie Phytologie Phytolisse Ultra Shine Smoothing Serum (Fabien Roussel), Kiehl's Crème with Silk Groom (Darin Birchler, who loves how it adds moisture and defines texture in dry, thick hair), and Paul Mitchell The Conditioner (a surprising choice for a styling product from Kathryn Alice). Two pros pick mousses: Danielle Browning (Prive Weightless Amplifier) and Nathaniel Hawkins (TRESemmé), who says, "More mousse is a good thing. Don't be afraid to use a lot. It's probably the most versatile styling product that allows you to create volume, body, or beautifully defined curls. TRESemmé Tres Mousse Extra Hold is an affordable classic." He also loves TRESemmé Tres Two Extra Hold Hair Spray: "It doesn't contain water so it never causes frizz or for the hairstyle to 'fall'." Two other star stylists pick hair sprays: Oribe (L'Oreal Elnett) and Ric Pipino (Kerastase). Pipino also chose his Pipino Flirt Flexible Hold Hair Gel.

Straightening and Curling Products

The Buzz from the Beauty Editor
I get a blow-out a couple of times a year. I like the occasional change, for a special occasion, and I like to see how long it's really gotten. The rest of the time, I don't bother. I live in Florida, and keeping naturally curly hair sleek and straight is a losing battle. These products

are designed to keep curly hair tamed and trouble-free. After applying a base of rich conditioners, I like to use one of the following products sparingly over the length of my hair to add definition and shine. My favorites are TIGI Bed Head Control Freak Frizz Control & Straightener Serum, $15.95, and Ouidad Climate Control Gel, $18.

What the Pros Choose

Some of the pros chose to play it straight, with smoothing products like TIGI Bed Head After-Party Smoothing Cream (Meg Thompson), Charles Worthington Results Relax and Unwind Blow Dry Straightening Balm (Charles Worthington), Phytotherathrie Phytodefrisant (Anthony Rocanello), and TRESemmé Anti-Frizz Styling Secret (Nathaniel Hawkins, who loves that it's affordable and not greasy). Kerastase Oleo-Relax is the smoothing choice for four experts: Jan Marini, Shauna Raisch, Ric Pipino, and Darin Birchler, who claims that half a pump of this coveted serum on towel-dried hair prior to blow-drying will ensure smooth, beautiful tresses. Wende Zomnir plays up her curls with Frédéric Fekkai Luscious Curls and Frédéric Fekkai Wave Creating Spray, while Barry Reitman prefers Graham Webb Intensives Making Waves Curl Defining Gel for his curly-haired clients because it's not stiff, dry, or flaky. Kattia Solano treats medium to thick curly hair with Kerastase Elasto-Curl Crème, a defining cream for thick or curly hair, and Shinbi Magic Move in Soft. Rachel Lindy chooses a few curl-enhancing products: Kerastase Elasto-Curl Weightless Mousse (for fine hair) and Defining Forming Crème (for thick hair), and the line of styling products from CurlFriends, especially the Replenishing Leave-In Conditioner and Rejuvenate Texturizing Mist. Other experts go for versatile, shine-enhancing products. Julie Hewett

chooses Bumble and bumble and Kerastase; Mala Elhassan picks Graham Webb Nolita Whipped Wax; June Jacobs goes for John Frieda and Yuki Systems; Meredith Green picks Pureology Shine Max; Oribe chooses his own Moisture Crème; and Dee DeLuca-Mattos chooses Ecru New York Silk Nectar Serum.

Groomers, Waxes, and Pomades

The Buzz from the Beauty Editor

I wash my hair every other day, so I rely on these products for between-shampoo touch-ups. They freshen, tame frizz, and add shine, making hair look just-washed and fabulous. No matter how thick or porous your hair is, go easy on these products. Apply just a little to begin with, and start at the ends. Any product that's left on your hands can be used to smooth out the top of your hair and the hairline. My favorites are Aveda Brilliant Anti-Humectant Pomade, $18, Kusco Murphy Lavender Hair Creme, $23.75, and Mario Russo Styling Creme, $24.50.

What the Pros Choose

Bumble and bumble turns up twice on this list, chosen by Julie Hewett and Darin Birchler (Sumotech—he loves how a dime-sized amount creates rugged texture in short hair). Kerastase also gets two nods: it is Hewett's second pick, and that of Shauna Raisch, who specifies the Lait Nutri-Sculpt. Other waxy wonders include Redken Smart Wax (Nelson Chan's pick), Sebastian Molding Mud (Dee DeLuca-Mattos), Robert Kree Mold It Molding Paste (Mala Elhassan), Murray's Original Pomade (Oribe and Anthony Rocanello), and Charles Worthington Dream Hair Perfect Reflection Texturising Wax (Charles

Worthington). Other picks include Paul Mitchell Super Skinny Serum (Barry Reitman), Aveda Light Elements Defining Whip (Wende Zomnir), Kerastase Nacre Nutri-Sculpt (Ric Pipino), and Phytotherathrie Phytodefrisant Botanical Relaxing Balm (Kathryn Alice, who loves that it won't weigh down fine hair).

Chapter Ten

Hair Apparent:
The Color Consultations

People make a lot of assumptions about us based on our hair color. As a brunette, people might assume that I'm smart and sophisticated. Or that I'm boring and stuffy. Blondes deal with their own assumptions. On the positive side, they are often perceived as sexy and sunny. The downside? Well, we've all heard the dumb-blonde jokes. Hair color instantly, overwhelmingly identifies us. It reveals something of our ethnic background, our personalities, even our character. Perhaps that's why choosing a colorist is one of the most important things you can do. A trained colorist can help you manipulate the image you send out to the world. After all, if people are going to make assumptions, at least make sure they assume the best.

THE 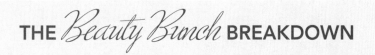 BREAKDOWN

Anthony Rocanello: senior colorist at Madison Avenue's Julien Farel Salon in New York City.

Louis Viél: passionate hair colorist and co-owner of Manhattan's Miano Viél Salon, Viél's celebrity-client list includes Heidi Klum, Melanie Griffith, and Melina Kanakaredes.

Beth Minardi: one of America's leading hair color authorities, and co-owner with husband Carmine of New York City's Minardi Salon. Minardi counts

celebrities like Cameron Diaz, Christie Brinkley, Faye Dunaway, Brad Pitt, Matt Dillon, Sarah Jessica Parker, and Mandy Moore as her clients.

Barry Reitman: star hairstylist with over twenty-five years of experience serving an exclusive clientele of celebrities and royalty.

Linda Deslauriers: founder of Hair Garden, a holistic hair company based in Hawaii and Los Angeles, and the author of an upcoming hair-care book.

Reynald Ricard: top colorist and co-owner of the trendy Red Market Salon and Lounge in New York City who has worked with celebrities like Anne Heche and Sting.

Todd Fox: top colorist with Frédéric Fekkai Salon & Spa, New York City.

Rachel Lindy: stylist at Los Angeles's Trim Salon, and winner of *Allure*'s coveted Up and Coming Star Stylist award.

Spresa Bojkovic: hair colorist and owner of the Damian West Salon.

Diane Gardner: Hollywood hairstylist, colorist, and makeup artist known as the Makeover Specialist.

Kathryn Alice: beauty publicist with her own firm, the Alice Company.

Peter Lamas: founder and chairman of Lamas Beauty International, a rapidly growing, well-respected natural beauty product manufacturer.

David Cotteblanche: star stylist and co-owner of New York City's Red Market Salon and Lounge in the trendy Meatpacking district.

Michael O'Rourke: founder and master hairstylist of Sexy Hair Concepts.

Jessica Tingley: hair designer at Frédéric Fekkai Salon & Spa in Beverly Hills. Her work has graced celebrities such as Daisy Fuentes, Maggie Gyllenhaal, Mischa Barton, and Kerry Washington.

Damien Miano: celebrity hairstylist whose work has appeared in countless top magazines, including *Cosmopolitan*, *Glamour*, and *W*. Miano is the co-owner of New York City's hot Miano Viél Salon.

Ouidad: stylist, salon owner, educator, and author who has earned a respected reputation as the Curly Hair Expert.

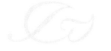

COLOR CONSULTATIONS

The Buzz from the Beauty Editor

Recently, I was distracted during my microdermabrasion treatment by the words on my esthetician's T-shirt: "Blondes are adored. Brunettes are ignored." While I didn't agree with the sentiment, the shirt does convey how strongly people identify with (and are identified by) their hair color. Hair color is one of the first things people notice about you, and it instantly conveys something about who you are and where you come from. Make sure it says what you want it to with these colorful tips from the pros.

Insider Information from the Beauty Bunch

Preventing Damage

"You should have a deep-conditioning treatment in the salon every time you have your hair colored. Don't be afraid that it's going to weigh down your hair. They are applied from the mid-shaft down. Also, using shampoos and conditioners designed specifically for color-treated hair makes a big difference." Louis Viél

Hair Herbs

"Brew an herbal tea, let it cool, and use it as a final leave-in hair rinse. Horsetail and nettle are great for all hair colors. Chamomile, lemon peel, rhubarb powder for blonde hair; sage, rosemary, lavender, and bay leaf for gray and dark hair; nettle and hibiscus flowers for red hair." Linda Deslauriers

Do It Yourself

"My advice for home color: if you choose a shade relatively close to your own natural color, you will be fine—as long as you follow the manufacturer's instructions. If you want a significant color change, or if your hair is very dark naturally, or if you have a relaxer or a perm—I *beg* you to see a colorist. *Please.* Also, if your hair is currently blonde, and you wish to deepen the hair back to brown, *please do not attempt this at home!*" Beth Minardi

Home Help

Home hair color "has its place in the world. There's a big market for it. If you don't have the time or a good salon nearby or the financial flexibility, there are ways to color at home. Always buy a shade lighter than you think you want, and leave it on for two-thirds of the time. Use a bunch of old towels. Don't do anything drastic. If you really want a major change, don't do it at home. Stick to minor changes. I'm not a big fan of at-home highlighting." Louis Viél

Born-with-It Beauty

"Hair color is makeup for the hair. Would someone walk out of the house without makeup? I doubt it. We can enhance what we have or maybe cover a little bit. I do a natural dimensional color that looks as if nature did it. If hair looks as if it's colored, then it's wrong. All I do is enhance it." Barry Reitman

Color-Coordinated

"Coordinate your wardrobe with your hair color. Take out your clothes and in front of a mirror, in a well-lit room, hold each piece close to your hair. See which colors make your hair stand out or which colors blend well with your hair. Eliminate the colors that overpower your hair or create an unfavorable contrast." Linda Deslauriers

BRUNETTES AND BRASSINESS

The Buzz from the Beauty Editor

If you're a brunette, like me, you know that the sun doesn't always bring out the best in your hair color. Here, the pros give you tips for bringing out the best in brown hair, and banishing brassiness.

Insider Information from the Beauty Bunch

Highlighting a Brunette

"I recommend doing some very soft highlights for the first time. On a brunette, you just want to go two to three shades lighter. Most brunettes don't want to see red in their hair. Brown hair has a lot of red pigments. You have to take the red pigment out and go up a couple of levels. You can neutralize the color afterwards with a gloss. The best way is to just apply the highlights and check them often and stop the process at the right time. If you go over the time, it's going to get too red or orange or yellow. You can also use oil color. Oil-based highlights will be very soft and have more control." Reynald Ricard

Brunette Boost

"The best advice I give brunettes is to opt for color placed in varying 'slashes' throughout the hair. Try to avoid 'all-over single-process' color, as the hair usually turns out too dark or turns red after a week or two." Beth Minardi

Sassy Not Brassy

"The brassiness happens at the ends of the hair. Every once in a while, with brunettes, you need to run the color through from root to end. You can't just do a root touch-up every time. And there have got to be equal components of ashen tone to whatever natural or golden tones you're putting in your formula. A colorist that's working with a brunette and the results are not coming up is working with the wrong formula. All brunettes have some red in their hair naturally. On some it's more visible, and on some it's not. The darker the color, naturally, the more red you will have. There is even some red if you use a certain amount of ash. It's physically, chemically impossible for a very dark-haired Asian or Hispanic woman who wants light brown hair to have no red. The stylist needs to tell you that it is not possible. You'd have to strip away all the natural color and put color back in, but it kills the hair. I take my cue from nature. Someone who has dark brown hair with a little bit of warmth in it looks good because that's the intended natural by-product of the lightening process. Women are more accepting of that now." Louis Viél

The War on Warmth

"Single-process color, if you are going lighter, means you're removing the existing color and replacing it with a different color. Hair is made up of blue, red, and yellow. You have to go through the warm tones to get to a new shade. Women in the Northeast never want to see red in brown or blonde hair, and anything warm to them is red. If you want to go far from your color, and don't want to see coppers or bronze or red, then you'll have to bleach it out through the warmth, which is very damaging, time-consuming, and expensive. Sometimes, celebs do have some brassiness, but they are kindly lit. They're lit from above. Unless you are walking around with a spotlight over your hair, you're not going to look like that. If you want hair that's easier to maintain, you're going to have to pay for it with a little bit of warmth, but it will cost you less time and money." Todd Fox

Beautifying Brown

"The best way to begin infusing red tones into brown hair is for the colorist to alternately 'weave,' 'slash,' and 'slice' several tones of red, and red-brown, into the hair. This gives the brown hair a noticeable population of varying red and 'reddish' tones—and makes it very sexy, multi-dimensional, and interesting." Beth Minardi

Brown It Down

"For brunettes, make a pot of coffee, *sans* milk or sugar. Run it through your dry hair before you shampoo. Let it stand for three minutes and then use John Frieda Brilliant Brunette Shampoo to finish this treatment. This prevents oxidation to your hair. You should not do this more than once a week." Anthony Rocanello

Un-Brassy Brunette

"Highlights on brunettes are the most difficult. Most colorists don't get it. Blonde highlights are a lot easier. The only way to avoid brassy highlights in brown hair is to actually lighten the hair more than you want to. When brown hair lightens, it doesn't lighten to a pretty color. It goes through a few different shades: red, orange, and then gold. You have to use bleach on brown hair to get highlights. First, you bleach it past the red and orange until it is yellow, and then you add the color that you want. You have to make the color. Put a color gloss over it and create the tone that you want in the hair. I've mastered it by doing my own hair, but nobody else gets my hair color right. Get another application of color gloss toner between color appointments. Redken Shades are beautiful toners. One day in the sun and the toner will come right out of your hair, so have it done regularly. And prevent fading by wearing a hat." Rachel Lindy

GOODBYE GRAY

The Buzz from the Beauty Editor
Prematurely gray hair runs in my family, and unfortunately, it didn't skip me. I've been coloring my hair for five years, and I'm only thirty-six. That's why I grilled the pros for their top gray-eliminating tips. My hope is that you'll find them as useful as I have.

Insider Information from the Beauty Bunch

Pigment Perfection
"Everyone's hair color starts with two primary pigments: red and brown. It either has less or more of these two colors. If you get gray, and your hair color is in the medium to dark range, it will get reddish or lighter. It's a loss of pigment." Barry Reitman

Disguising Your Gray
How often you need a salon touch-up "all depends on your percentage of gray. Color can be done between four to eight weeks, but the average is every four to six weeks. Once you've reached your desired color goal, there's no reason to color all the way to the ends every time. Only color the roots. At every third color [appointment], it is good to run the color all the way through to keep the hair color even. This is because the ends of hair oxidize, which means that they lighten or get brassy." Spresa Bojkovic

Gray Gauge
"Identify the percentage of gray and determine whether the color is permanent or semipermanent. If the hair is under twenty-five percent gray, you don't want permanent color. You want the gray to look like highlights." Louis Viél

Goodbye Gray
"To cover gray in the most modern way, especially with brunettes, I recommend using a non-ammonia 'demi' color, in a salon—*not* at home. Choose a tone *slightly* lighter and *slightly* warmer than the natural brown, and apply to scalp area only—then less time on the ends and hair shaft." Beth Minardi

Shades of Gray
"Semipermanent color will not cover gray; it just blends and mutes it. To completely cover gray hair, you have to use permanent color." Barry Reitman

Downplay the Gray
"Changing where you part your hair can help if there is more gray hair in one spot (i.e., if most of your

gray is in the middle, switch to a side part). Bangs also help if you have grays framing your face. Another good trick is to add highlights; they help to camouflage grays." Spresa Bojkovic

The Perfect Match

"The best way to match your hair color when concealing gray hair is to go to a professional for a color consultation. At home, if you're unsure of which color matches best, I always think it's better to go a shade lighter than darker. Lighter will not only cover the gray but will blend more like highlights, while the darker shade will look like a halo where applied." Spresa Bojkovic

Gray Guidance

"You can do mostly one shade of single process for someone that has gray and wants to cover it. If you have just a few grays, a coloring shampoo can cover the gray a little, but with more gray, you need to use something stronger, like a single process. You can usually come in every four to five weeks to cover gray, but sometimes it can be two weeks. It depends on your expectations. Some people don't want to see any gray." Reynald Ricard

Goodbye Gray

"Permanent hair color covers gray, and you need to go back every four to five weeks for maintenance. Semipermanent will blend gray and coat it, and it fades off in six to eight weeks." Todd Fox

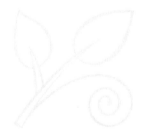

COLOR ERRORS

The Buzz from the Beauty Editor

When I was a senior in high school, I went with a group of friends to see *The Witches of Eastwick*. My crush kept commenting on Susan Sarandon's gorgeous red, curly hair, so I went out and bought a box of home hair color and dyed my hair auburn. At first, the difference was minimal, and no one noticed, but by spring, I was officially a redhead. Worse, my crush had ended. I took myself to the local salon for a quick fix, and emerged as a Goth, with pitch-black hair. That's the last time I attempted to color my own hair. Read on for other, not-so-obvious color disasters.

Insider Information from the Beauty Bunch

Tone Deaf

The most common mistake is using the "wrong color for their pigmentation. You have to take into consideration the color of the skin and the eyes, and the look of a person. You can have the most beautiful color and beautiful clothes, but if it doesn't go with your pigmentation, it doesn't enhance the color of your eyes or skin. Like if you see a platinum blonde who would look better and softer with soft highlights. If you want to go extreme, you have to have an extreme attitude and color; you can't go soft and classic. Someone who can go platinum blonde will often also look very good with dark hair colors because they have cool tones." Reynald Ricard

Contrasting Colors

"The number-one hair color mistake that I see is when there is no contrast between hair and skin color. Everyone does it, and it's the worst thing you can do, because it makes you look average. If the hair is light brown and the skin is yellow-toned, from a distance, you will look all beige, all one tone. Celebs are always striking, because there is an extreme contrast between their skin and hair. An African American woman with blonde hair, or cherry-colored hair, is so striking, because the contrast is so great. If you see someone really tan with blonde hair, or pale with black hair, that's striking, because the contrast of the hair against the skin makes them look strikingly beautiful." Diane Gardner

Going Goth

"The worst mistake a colorist can make is to color the hair too dark. It's also the most difficult to correct. If you want your hair to be medium chestnut brown and you come away with your hair dyed black, that's the biggest problem." Louis Viél

Catastrophic Color

"You see too many clients who are going too far from their natural color, like dark brown to blonde, or medium brown to light blonde. Going the farthest from the natural hair color, on the lighter side, doesn't work at all. The farther you get from nature, the worse it looks. It doesn't go with your skin color. And they don't prepare for the maintenance. Nothing is worse than going too far from the natural spectrum and not maintaining it. That looks atrocious. A lot of colorists will take your money, give you what you want, send you out of there, and don't care if they see you again. That's why clients hop from chair to chair. They're running around frustrated, looking for someone to help them fix it. Stick to something closer to what nature has given you." Todd Fox

REDHEADS AND BLONDES

The Buzz from the Beauty Editor

Redheads and blondes have unique hair-coloring needs. For blondes, the goal is to make hair look multidimensional, sophisticated, and healthy, as if it grew out of your head that way. Redheads want their color to be rich, deep, and never brassy. Read on as the pros show you how to get the color you want.

Insider Information from the Beauty Bunch

Ravishing Red

"The single process that's most often done for someone who doesn't necessarily need it done is usually in the red family. To establish a red that has depth or brightness at the same time, you have to make a commitment to it. You can't just do highlights." Louis Viél

Blonde Ambition

"Often we hear that as we get older, we should go blonde. It's a bunch of [garbage]. The only reason that is said is that when hair is gray, it's devoid of color, and blonde has more longevity, in terms of roots. You don't see black and white. When we lose color from our hair, we lose it from our skin. But without anything reflecting onto the face, you look washed out. For a very fair blonde who's older, there's no contrast, so she has to wear a lot of make-up to have some definition. Nothing is reflecting color onto the skin. Not everyone has the skintone to pull it off. You want something to flatter your skin so you can wear minimal makeup. Don't stray from what nature gave you. Go one level lighter or darker than your natural color. If your hair was white, go to what you had when you were younger. There are no mistakes in nature. What you were given is always the best." Todd Fox

Radical Red
"Redheads are my specialty. That's what I'm known for. Reds are divided into two categories: blue-based reds and orange-based reds. Orange-based reds are the most natural; no one is born with a blue-based red. But orange-based reds are not the best look for you if are milky white with freckles. More of a blonde would be pretty. On darker olive skin, a blue-red is better, but not a wine or magenta or fuchsia unless you're seventeen and in a band. You can temper orange-based red with blonde or brown hair to get a softer tone or a deeper, richer shade. Blue-based reds tend to be a little more surreal. On dark hair with [an] olive complexion, it may be very pretty to do a wine color. It's not natural but it's still pretty. It doesn't have to look natural to look good. What is natural is what's on your head and obviously you want to change that, so just because it doesn't look natural doesn't mean it can't be beautiful. You can't get hung up on the semantics. Go for what looks best." Louis Viél

Battling the Brassies
"There are a couple of shampoos out there that tend to be effective for getting rid of brassiness. Clairol ShimmerLights Bluing Shampoo can remove brassiness from blonde hair." Louis Viél

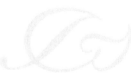

HIGHLIGHTING HELP

The Buzz from the Beauty Editor
There's quite a bit of controversy in this category between two opposing highlighting camps. On one side, you'll find the pros who use baliage, a method of freely painting highlights on the hair. They feel that seeing the color develop, rather than covering it with foil, gives them more control over the finished result. On the other side, there are the pros who prefer foils. Their argument is that foils are more precise and that they allow you to deposit color closer to the root. Whichever method your colorist chooses, highlighting is best left to a professional.

Insider Information from the Beauty Bunch

Picking Highlights
"I take my cue from the natural highlights in the hair. I'm not one of those colorists who says that if your eyes are blue, your hair should be blonde. I ask myself, *What do the natural hues of the hair lend themselves towards, golden or red?* Eye and skin color play a part. Color is a very individual, perceived thing, and it's very subjective. As a colorist with a trained eye, there are specifics so I'll be able to look at something and say this is golden or red and I'll know that's what it is. I typically only like women to bring in photos of themselves, maybe from the past. I like to see what they liked themselves to look like, not a picture of Julianne Moore's color, unless you don't have a picture with your color the way you like it. But pictures don't always print true to life. I like it if a client

says, 'I wore my hair darker in my twenties, and I think I like that better, but what do you think?' I don't like to show them a color chart. They don't know what they're looking at. I'm looking at five colors and know what they'll look like blended together, but clients can't really do that." Louis Viél

Highlight Help

"A lot of people do their highlights just on the roots when they grow out, and they don't apply it to the ends. Most of the time, you can do just the roots, because it's more difficult to apply it correctly on the ends, and make it look natural. On blondes, I do some thin and thick highlights and leave some space in between because it looks natural. Most of them come back every three months, and it looks good. It grows out nicely, and looks more natural. It's not so even and mechanical. You have to look at the whole picture on the canvas, and then you can just make some pieces lighter where you want them. You don't have to do too much to make a blonde beautiful. After a blonde is overprocessed, you have to do lowlights to make it better." Reynald Ricard

Highlighting Hint

"For hair highlights that won't show a line when they grow out, find a hairdresser who paints them on. A good colorist will follow the color lines each touchup, leaving the dark areas dark for a more natural-looking overall hair color effect. Indiscriminate foiling results in the bottom hair getting entirely bleached out with no darker color left." Kathryn Alice

Foil Fan

"The best method of highlighting hair is foils. I do not believe in painting hair, or baliage. It only looks good the first time on virgin hair. You don't get subtle or multitonal looks that way. You get closer to the root with foil, and you are really placing foils where you want to be in relation to the haircut. On every foil job, there's a different pattern that the foils go in. It's far more artistic to place foils in a pattern that's appropriate for the look you're trying to achieve. You can work with so many different colors." Louis Viél

Highlighting Methods

"Our salon is known for baliage [a technique where color is painted onto the hair], but depending on what kind of effect you are looking for, I might do baliage or foils. Baliage tends to look more blended than foils." Todd Fox

Technique Talk

"I paint. I don't use foil. I don't use any cover or plastic so I can see what is happening. If you use bleach to make the hair a bit brighter, it's difficult to control the process because it's inside the foil and you can't see it. When you paint it on, you see exactly what is going on and as soon as the color is right you rinse it and the color is perfect. When you use foil, it's hard to color the same pieces you did before, but with painting or baliage, you can see it and do the same pieces you did before. If you use cotton or plastic, it's the same as with the foil. What is important is to be able to see the whole picture." Reynald Ricard

GOODBYE GREEN

The Buzz from the Beauty Editor

Jokes are made about blue-haired old ladies, but few comedians comment on the prevalence of blondes with a greenish cast. For the unfortunate bearer of this hair color, it's no joke. The combination of chlorine and hair bleach is not a pretty one. Fortunately, the pros know how to treat and prevent it.

Insider Information from the Beauty Bunch

The Green-Haired Monster

"Chlorine in the water makes hair turn green. To avoid this, before you go in the pool, protect your hair with some oil or something to close the cuticle so that the water doesn't penetrate into your hair and change the pigmentation. This only happens in someone who is very blonde and overprocessed, because the cuticle gets so porous." Reynald Ricard

The Green Culprit

"Green hair only really happens if your hair is very blonde and you spend a lot of time in chlorine. Don't go into the hot tub, and ask your stylist for something to protect your hair." Louis Viél

Green Be Gone

"For blondes who develop unwanted green: The green is usually a stain which shows on the lightened hair. Often, it is copper, which oxidizes greenish from chlorinated water or treated water running through copper-lined pipes. Several great salon products have been designed to 'chelate,' or 'lift,' the green from the hair. Green also happens when hair has been bleached—or lightened—too much. A color-enhancing shampoo in a golden or gold/orange shade will softly and safely neutralize this color. This shampoo *must* be custom-blended by a colorist in a salon selling custom-blended color-enhancing shampoos." Beth Minardi

LENGTHS AND EXTREMES

The Buzz from the Beauty Editor

I recently spotted a woman with neon-bright red hair in a choppy, mid-length style, and had to hold myself back. I so desperately wanted to approach her and ask her what she was thinking. Extreme colors are hard to pull off, and the pros agree that they require a short cut and equally extreme overall look.

Insider Information from the Beauty Bunch

Starry Eyed

"With some stars, like Jennifer Lopez, the lighter shades work on them, but these are women who do not get ready themselves. They have someone on hand to smooth their hair, blow it out, make sure the part is in the right place to make their highlights like that. Your hair can look overprocessed, fuzzy, and dirty [if you go for extreme color], and you'll see the roots if it's not styled properly. You have to commit to the whole look, like Gwen Stefani. Her makeup always suits her look perfectly. You need to pull off the whole look when you are going extreme with your color. Our salon [Frédéric Fekkai] tends to be a little more classic." Todd Fox

Length and Color

"I don't think length determines color except for the extremes. If you want very light blonde hair or bright red or really, really dark hair, extremes of anything, those look best on short haircuts. As soon as you involve length with extreme color, the darkest colors can look helmet-y and the lightest colors can look strawlike. Multi-tonal looks are key with long hair. Solid colors can give a rock-and-roll look to short hair." Louis Viél

Extreme Options
"Platinum blonde is better on short hair. Some reds are better on short hair. Mostly, I don't like to see a white blonde with long hair. A uniform single-process bleach blonde is much better on short hair." Reynald Ricard

Going Extreme
"The one thing I will say is that I love to do extreme changes and lots of women can look great in lots of different colors, but there are very, very few Madonnas in the world, very few human chameleons. She has a look, a style, a character, that can morph into these various different looks. Hair color is the first thing people see. If your hair color is terrible, people are going to see that first. It doesn't matter that you're wearing Harry Winston diamonds and a Roberto Cavalli dress and your figure is fabulous. There are very few women that look good in all extremes. Geena Davis pulls it off; Lindsay Lohan does not." Louis Viél

The Long and the Short of It
"With a short, edgy cut, the cut should stand alone, and color should enhance the cut. You can't battle the color against the cut. Something is going to lose. For Vidal Sassoon's cuts, or on Isabella Rosellini, the cut stood by itself. There's more freedom with short hair, more freedom with hair color as far as fashion shades, like bright copper, stop-sign reds. If you put those on long hair, they look witchy and unsophisticated. Longer hair should be softer. You want it to look as healthy as possible and to keep as many chemicals off of it as possible. There's nothing worse than long hair that's damaged. That bothers me, and these are the women you see who always have their hair pulled back. There's this identity thing with long hair. Women in their forties and fifties are pushing the envelope with long hair. You see women walking down Madison Avenue with long hair, stilettos, and tight pants, and when they turn around they look like the Cryptkeeper. It's an individual thing, whether or not to keep your hair long. But I have yet to figure out why women hold on to long hair that they pull back." Todd Fox

TECHNICAL TALK

The Buzz from the Beauty Editor
Hair color can be baffling. If your colorist gives you a choice of permanent and semi-permanent color, you need to know the difference. This brief hair-color course will give you the scoop on the different types of hair color, so you and your colorist can pick the one that most suits your needs.

Insider Information from the Beauty Bunch

Choosing a Technique
"It depends on the motivation for color. Is it to cover gray, or to accent natural color? You're either making a color change or accenting what's already there. Most women don't want to do a single-process hair color unless they absolutely despise their own color: if it's mousy or dishwater blonde or very dull, or they have gray, or they want a complete departure. Single-process is more maintenance, so unless

there's a reason to do it, think twice. You might want to highlight your hair instead. It's more expensive and time-consuming in the salon, but you come a lot less often." Louis Viél

Water Worries

"If you have well water, not city water, it will be high in mineral content. A lot of highlights tend to look green or blue from too much copper and iron in the water. If there is any residue in your toilet or sink, you might have water that's high in mineral content. You may want to avoid pale shades if you have that kind of water and no softener in the system. I see clients from Connecticut or Pennsylvania with this problem. You can feel it in the hair. You may also expect your color to fade more quickly." Todd Fox
[Note: Combat the harsh mineral effects of your water with one of the new water filters that attach to your showerhead, like the Jonathan Product Beauty Water Shower Purification System.]

Carefree Color

"Single-process color requires less maintenance than highlights. The same shade all over your head can warm or lighten your hair up a bit. Semipermanent color is much more subtle, but permanent color is the only thing that will lighten the hair and cover gray. Once you achieve the color that you want, you can just have permanent color applied to the roots and a use a conditioning color gloss on the rest of the hair." Rachel Lindy

Comprehending Color

"Don't go too far away from your natural color or you will see the fade off. The only thing permanent about permanent hair color is that it permanently gets rid of your natural hair color. Semipermanent color actually lasts longer, because it fades more gradually, so that's your pick if you want less maintenance. Often, clients will think the color fell off the hair, when it really just grew in. Single-process is more of a commitment, because you never see your actual color." Todd Fox

Color Definition

"There are two main choices in hair color: permanent or semipermanent. For permanent hair color, the color is mixed with peroxide, which opens up the cuticle shaft and enables the color to go inside the hair. Semipermanent color has no lifting properties. It stays on the outside of the hair and washes off with time. There are no real roots with semipermanent color because it fades gradually; with permanent color you will see your roots as it grows out." Barry Reitman

Curly Color

"With hair that is a little bit curly, I do the ends lighter. I tease the hair very extreme, then just apply the bleach or color with my hands. If you tease your hair, the color doesn't touch all the hair; it touches only some of the ends." Reynald Ricard

The Goods on Gloss

"If you don't use a gloss, the color will change for the better, and get lighter in a nice way. If you go in the sun and the hair gets lighter naturally, the color is nice and natural. It's the same process with colored hair if the process is stopped when the color is perfect. But a gloss means you want to fix something. A lot of colorists do a gloss to fix a mistake if they go too light or too red or go too long with the foils. You see all these girls on the streets with very light highlights on the roots and the ends are brassy, and there's no shine or freshness." Reynald Ricard

Coloring Curls

"I've developed a very specific highlighting technique for curly hair called Curlights. I've been highlighting Melina Kanakaredes for ten years, and we straighten her hair first before we highlight it. We might even flatiron it first. This is for curly-haired women who wear their hair curly all the time." Louis Viél

COLOR COMMUNICATION

The Buzz from the Beauty Editor
Color is a very difficult thing to communicate, because one word can mean different things to different people. That's why I think a picture is essential. Otherwise, you might ask for caramel and end up with honey.

Insider Information from the Beauty Bunch

Great Expectations
"The biggest thing with the client is to build a relationship with the colorist, and work towards something with them. It might take more than one visit. A disaster that didn't happen overnight can't be repaired overnight. There are no quick fixes in hair color. It generally takes as long to get hair back into a good condition as it did to get it into a bad condition. Many women change their hair with big life changes, like divorce, infidelity, the kids going off to school. They rip pictures out of magazines. In their minds, they think if we take them from boring brown to blonde, they'll look like Heidi Klum. It can help, but they need to have reasonable expectations. We're not going to solve their problems. [Another problem is] clients thinking they can go full spectrum and then back, like blonde in summer and red in fall. We see

stars and celebrities go through this, but we don't realize how much time went by between a star's hair color in a movie and when you see them in *US Weekly*. It's very damaging. They're not prepared to get haircuts. There's no way to do it without damage. Pick something that works for you, and don't go too far from what's natural. But if your hair is short, and you have the time and money, go for it." Todd Fox

Clear Consultation
"Clients should stay away from trying to use the lingo. Speak in lay terms, and be as clear as possible. I just need to see what you're looking for. The consultation is really important with the colorist. I have to know why you don't like it and what you don't like and what you mean when you say you don't like anything red. 'My mother used to dye her hair red, and I don't want my hair to look like that.' That's the key with everything, having a real clear-cut consultation and finding out what they like and don't like about their hair at that moment." Louis Viél

Color Coded
"It's so difficult for a hairdresser or a client to describe a hair color. How do you describe a color? A beige might be a wheat shade or there may be some gold. So it's important, if you're going for a specific color, to come in with a picture. I once had a woman bring in a huge 11" x 14" frame because she liked the hair color of the woman in the picture that came with the frame. So bring in a picture, and then the stylist should look at your hair color, your skin color, and start from there. A surefire way is to take a swatch of hair color and put it next to the woman's skin, and if it looks good on her skin or with her eyes, it's a winner. I don't veer too far off from her natural color. But if she wants to go from dark to blonde, she'll have to understand the maintenance involved. She'll need to come in every four weeks.

Hair frames your face. It's really important. You have to enhance your own natural beauty." Barry Reitman

Three Options

"My theory on offering color to clients is that I believe in good, better, best. You should be able to offer each client three different options, all presumably better than what it looks like when they walk in the salon. Very often, that is linked to the amount of time and money they are going to spend on their hair. A single-process color might look good, and highlights will look better, and the best might be to do both. How much time do you have to put into it, and how much money? It all falls under lifestyle. If you have the lifestyle, time, energy, and money to devote to your look, then go for it." Louis Viél

Find Your Frequency

"Many factors determine how often a client should come in: the texture, hairstyle, et cetera. If your hair is fine or straight with a part, you're going to see roots more quickly than on thick and curly hair with no part. A lot depends on texture, the amount of gray, and the level of contrast between the natural color and the hair color choice. You can get away with a single-process every three to six weeks, and highlights between six to ten weeks." Louis Viél

COLOR-CONSCIOUS SHAMPOOS

The Buzz from the Beauty Editor

Even though my hair is a dark brown, my hair color tends to get brassy, turning almost orange at the ends if I neglect it long enough. Once, on a whim, I bought a bottle of a coloring shampoo designed for use on black hair, hoping it would counteract the orange. Instead, it created a black and orange mess better suited for Halloween than Hollywood. I learned that, in most matters of hair color, it's wise to seek professional advice, but sometimes even the pros don't agree. While they universally stressed the importance of a good shampoo for color-treated hair, things got controversial when talk turned to pigmented shampoos. Even the pros who like these shampoos agree that you need to choose wisely, and enlist the help of your colorist.

Insider Information from the Beauty Bunch

Shampoo Strategies

"Some [pigment shampoos], like ARTec, are good. They have a good amount of pigment. At the same time, you need to know which tone to use for your complexion. It can sometimes neutralize the highlights. After two to three weeks, if your color is not as shiny, you can use a pigment shampoo. Ask your colorist which shampoo will match your color. I have customers who have beautiful highlights, then use a pigment shampoo and the highlights disappear. Mix pigment with your regular shampoo. It's even more effective than a color shampoo. It gives more pigment and shine. Try Clairol Jazzing for highlights. You can use it every two weeks, and it keeps the color fresh. It's like a gloss application at [a] salon. A good shampoo is key to keeping color fresh." Reynald Ricard

Shampoo Specifics

"I recommend a color shampoo to keep color from fading, and it can alter your color slightly. ARTec's color shampoos are good. If you're a blonde, and your color is too white, Lemon Flower will make it warmer. If you'd like your blonde to be more golden, use Sunflower, which is the prettiest. It's my favorite warm golden shade. Apply a color shampoo after your regular shampoo. It should not be used in place of a regular shampoo because it doesn't have the same function; it's just to deposit color." Rachel Lindy

Color Care

"Pick a shampoo for color-treated hair. Don't pay three hundred dollars for hair color and then use Pantene. Invest in a shampoo and conditioner made for color-treated hair, that's pH balanced. Use a sun-protectant styling product or a hat. Wear a bathing cap. Take your suntan lotion and use it to slick your hair back. The same thing that protects your body is going to protect your hair. The best thing after swimming is to shampoo immediately. Wash your hair before you get in, put conditioner in it, and then as soon as you get out, shampoo. This will often stop the green or bleaching from the pool. Don't burn hair with too much heat while blow-drying it. Flatirons are a no-no as much as possible. It makes color fade. Leave it to the professionals." Todd Fox

Color-Conscious Shampoos

"Anything that can cause a buildup on the hair can eventually dull the hair. Shampoos and conditioners designed to be gentle to color-treated hair are important, but I'm not a big fan of the coloring shampoos. If your color is being done properly, it should not fade in between appointments." Louis Viél

Color Care

"Hair-care companies are making shampoos and conditioners that help keep your color from fading and protect the integrity of the hair. You should not invest money in coloring your hair and then not invest in keeping it up." Rachel Lindy

SALON STRATEGIES

The Buzz from the Beauty Editor

We've all been there, sitting defenseless in a stylist's chair and failing to speak up. Once, as a well-meaning but inexperienced stylist started to *tease* my thick, curly hair in preparation for a black-tie event, I burst into tears. I resolved then and there to speak up. I got up out of that chair, washed my own hair, and styled it as usual. If you pick a top stylist, you will probably never experience this type of drama, but it's still important to learn how to communicate and convey your vision for your hair. A good stylist will insist on it.

Insider Information from the Beauty Bunch

Speak Up

"The key between a stylist and a client is communication, and I really think that's up to the hairdresser. It's very important for a top expert stylist to be able to communicate with the customer. That's what they are there for. The top stylists talk to their clients. This is what differentiates them from the rest. You have to get a feeling for what they want, what they're comfortable with, what kind of job they have, what is going to work for them at home. I know the hair, but I don't know the person. It is my job to open the lines of communication. Many times the client doesn't know what she wants; she just wants to be beautiful. It's my job to tell them how to get there." Barry Reitman

Stylist Splurge
"It's worth it to go to a popular, expensive hairdresser who will take your face shape into consideration. A good hairstylist is usually someone you read about in the paper or in fashion magazines. If you're in a state without star stylists, find someone who has a great haircut and ask them who cuts their hair." Diane Gardner

Honesty Counts
"Be very up-front and honest about what you want, and unless you've been going to the stylist for ten years, never say, 'Just do what you think is best.'" Peter Lamas

Show and Tell
"The stylist is supposed to communicate with the customer. The best way is to bring a picture and show him the style or color that you want." David Cotteblanche

Speak Easy
"Find a stylist that you can communicate with. If they have an attitude, get up and go. How are you going to explain your life and your feelings if the stylist's not listening? Some of them feel they are big shots and they don't listen. You are spending good money. They need to ask questions about your lifestyle, how you maintain your hair, do you have kids, how much time are you willing to devote to it,

and whether you are self-conscious about your nose or ears or the wrinkles on your brows. If he doesn't listen, he is an absolute idiot. He needs to know what to do to make your life easier so that you can maintain that haircut. Truthfully, you are designing a complete lifestyle. It's important for your hair to fit your schedule, the way you look, and how professional or athletic you are." Michael O'Rourke

Know It All
"I am open to being shown pictures of a hairstyle by a client, because then I get an idea what they want, and we can work towards it. My pet peeve is when a client has no idea what she wants, and then keeps changing her mind. Fortunately, most clients are pretty easy to work with." Jessica Tingley

Speak Out
"Be opinionated abut what you want, and hopefully understand your hair well enough to know what it will or won't do. I don't mind when people say exactly what they want. Either that, or just leave it to the stylist. You can say, 'I would like long or short, but I'll leave it to you to do the best thing.' But being in the middle is what drives a stylist crazy. That's when there's a breakdown of communication. When the client says, 'Do what you want, but not this or that.' Sometimes I want to pick up the scissors and comb and hand it to them and say, 'Maybe you can do it, because you've just tied my hands.' If you are very direct with what you want, that's wonderful. I don't mind if you show photographs, so I can see whether you're in left field. Bring in something visible or tangible if it looks like it could be your hair type. Be specific, be daring, be creative. You can give parameters. For example, you can say, 'I don't want short layers.' If you have no idea what you want, you should set up a time for a consultation with the stylist so you don't take up the time for your haircut. If

you go in completely unaware of what you want, that will require a ten-minute conversation, which will stress out the stylist." Damien Miano

Wash Not
"If you walk into a salon for the first time and your hair is shampooed before the stylist ever sees you, that's a definite get up and leave. Just walk out. A stylist simply can't tell what they are dealing with unless they see your hair dry. For example, with a long-haired client who wants to keep the length but to do something different at the same time, I will outline her haircut when the hair is dry. If the hair was wet, it would appear longer and we might end up taking too much off. When we've communicated and decided what length we want the hair, then we shampoo." Barry Reitman [Note: The only time this rule may not apply is with curly hair. See Ouidad's tip, below.]

Natural Woman
"If you have curly hair, your stylist should see your hair in its natural state, so the consultation should come after your hair has been shampooed. That's the best way to see it as it really is, because every time you style your hair, or pull it back, or up, you are creating an artificial curl wave. It's essential to see the curl the way it grows naturally." Ouidad

Staking a Stylist
"I recommend choosing a curly-haired stylist if you have curly hair. Curly hair has a mind of its own, and a stylist who has curly hair understands it. That is at least fifty percent of the battle. There's a comprehension of the way the hair works. The next thing I think you should do is to start slow with your stylist. Have a thorough conversation. Not a consultation, when the stylist is talking at you, but a back-and-forth conversation. Question. Debate. Have them explain what they are saying. Make sure you understand

their terminology, and that they understand yours. This discussion should last at least five minutes, and that's a long time. Then start with something simple, like a trim. Test out the stylist before you commit to having something major done to your hair." Ouidad

Style Speak
"Communication is so important. A stylist should be able to tell you which brushes to use and which products to use. You need to learn from [hello]. You are paying him good money to do your hair and part of that is maintaining it. It's no good if you walk out and it's great, but you can't do it again. If a client is educated, she will have all the tools and can do her hair in a short time." Michael O'Rourke

Clear Communication
"Make sure that you are clear in your discussion with your stylist; many clients don't explain what they want properly. At the same time, it's the stylist's job to ask the right questions and to make sure that they understand what you are asking for. It's not the client's job to know the terminology. But be as clear as you can. If you want your hair to frame your face, say that, or say that you want little pieces cut around your face. Don't say that you want your hair cut at an angle, which doesn't work for curly hair. The right words are important. The stylist should try to make sure that you know what you are saying, because it's not the client's job to understand the terms. Don't hesitate to really assert yourself to the stylist. A good stylist will not be offended." Ouidad

Prescriptive Products
"Your stylist should advise you on what products to use, when to use them, and when to switch. If it's humid in the summer and not in the winter, then you can't be applying the same products year round. You cannot apply hair products as a routine. It's not like

brushing your teeth. A lot of women consistently do the same thing every day, whether or not they need to. It shouldn't be an automatic shampoo-conditioner every day. It's prescriptive. I often won't put any moisturizer—conditioner—in the hair if it doesn't need it. You wouldn't take medicine consistently for something that is cleared up. You should base your hair care on the condition of your hair that day. If you come in with a dry scalp and dry ends, and the stylist recommends a product for that, then at some point your hair is going to be better. So you won't need to use the same product anymore. It should be about prescription hair health." Barry Reitman

Stylist Alert

A stylist should look first at your "face shape, hair texture, and frizz. And then what you want to do with your hair." Damien Miano

Personality First

"A stylist should take your personality into account. That's extremely important. He should enhance it, make it fun, or whatever you want to project. If you're feminine, maybe he can put some rollers in it and make you look like Marilyn Monroe. Every woman wants to be beautiful and wants to feel as sexy as possible. As an artist, the stylist should keep that in mind and bring out as much femininity as possible in the hair. He needs to bring that inside feeling out." Michael O'Rourke

Consult Your Stylist

"You can tell the personality and the style of the woman when she comes in. A stylist should ask what she does in her life. The main question is what she does to her hair. What kind of quality is there to the hair? She might have a blow-dry, but we wash her hair and it's curly. What kind of products do we use? Some women know what they want. The consulta-

tion is very important. It's eighty percent of the haircut. It's a big part of the job." David Cotteblanche

PRODUCT FILES

Post-Color Treatments

The Buzz from the Beauty Editor

My hair is long and naturally dry, but I used to keep it in pretty good condition because I never exposed it to heat or chemicals. It was "virgin" hair. But now that I'm forced to color it to cover gray, keeping it healthy takes a little more work. The night before I get my hair colored, I wash it, coat it with a deep conditioner, and then put it up or in a couple of braids. I look like Pippi Longstocking when I show up at the salon the next day, but the damage it saves my hair is worth it. Plus, the braids keep my hair untangled. Otherwise, by the time my colorist finishes concealing my roots, my hair is one big, frizzy, tangled mess. The pros have their own ideas about keeping colored hair in great condition.

What the Pros Choose

The pros have specific strategies for treating colored hair. For Anthony Rocanello and Reynald Ricard, Phyto products do the trick. Rocanello suggests this post-color strategy: "When you get home from the salon after having your color done, you can maintain it by using Phytotherathrie Phytojoba Shampoo if your hair is dry. Shampoo your hair until you get the bubbles working, and then let it sit for five minutes. Rinse it out and use Phytotherathrie Phytosésame Conditioner. Then use a hot towel on your hair to dry it. Apple cider vinegar hair baths are best for those summer buildups. This is great for blondes and redheads. Then use Phytotherathrie Phytolactum Shampoo and Phytotherathrie Phytobaume Conditioner to finish this treatment. This will help your hair in the summer heat." Ricard's options range from low-tech oil treatments to high-tech ionic treatments: "A hair mask or oil can treat damage caused by hair color. We can also do an ionic treatment at the salon. We have this process that will bring back fifty times more moisture to the hair. Phytotherathrie Phytonectar Ultra Nourishing Oil Treatment is also very good for hair repair." Nick Arrojo prefers the Wella Color Preserve line for its comprehensive color care. "Not only is the performance excellent," he says, "but they also protect your color from fading in the sun while giving your hair extra protection, shine, and support." The line includes a full range of shampoos, conditioners, and styling products.

Hair Color

The Buzz from the Beauty Editor

When your hair is long, thick, and curly, and the only reason you color is to cover gray, hair color appointments are a dreaded necessity rather than a luxury. I don't color my hair for fun. That's why I love the suggestions in this section. When you choose the best brands of hair color, and then maintain your hair in between appointments with products designed to cover gray, you can prolong the time between color appointments, saving time and money.

What the Pros Choose

The pros have very specific ideas about the best brands of hair color. For Louis Viél, the classics are still the best: "Wella is my favorite brand of hair color. Professionally, they are the best. After twenty years, the best brands are still Wella, Clairol, and L'Oreal." Reynald Ricard bases his brand choices on the specific application: "L'Oreal is one of my favorite brands of hair color, but I use different products for different processes. For a blonde to go to brunette, I use Young Color by Revlon. The color sticks on the hair and doesn't wash out. I also like Majorelle and Jacolore, and sometimes, Phyto."

Concealing gray hair is never fun, but fortunately, companies are coming out with quick, innovative ways to disguise roots between appointments, from temporary color washes to hair mascaras. The key is to not use anything that can permanently alter your color. Giella offers this suggestion: "Try using a non-permanent hair tint that washes out with shampoo. At GIELLA, we can custom-blend a hair tint that you brush on your roots with a mascara-type wand. It's a great way to get rid of gray hairs or add a little more blonde or copper at a moment's notice. It dries quickly and doesn't smudge." For Spresa Bojkovic, a product called ColorMark does the trick. "Brown hair with gray in it is covered most easily. ColorMark is an instant temporary hair color that not only covers gray professionally, but washes out when you shampoo, so that you are not compromising your professional color."

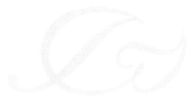

Chapter Eleven

Meticulous Manicures and Pedicures:
Get Groomed with Guidelines for Beautiful Hands and Fabulous Feet

Manicures and pedicures are an essential element of good grooming, as scruffy cuticles and scaly soles can ruin an otherwise immaculate appearance. No matter how much attention I've paid to the rest of my look, I don't feel polished unless my fingertips are. And men notice hands, too. My dad always compliments my mom on her pedicures, and though my husband never comments on my lipstick, he's the first to notice if my nails are chipped. Nothing is more flagrantly feminine than beautiful hands and feet. And though you may have to work hard at achieving glorious hair and stunning skin, it's relatively easy to treat yourself to a manicure or pedicure.

THE *Beauty Bunch* BREAKDOWN

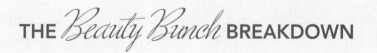

Elisa Ferri: celebrity manicurist affiliated with Nailene nail-care products, and author of *Style on Hand: Perfect Nail and Skincare*.

Giella: professional makeup artist and founder of GIELLA Custom Blend Cosmetics.

Peter Thomas Roth: skin-care entrepreneur with an eponymous skin-care line.

Dee Pearn: celebrity manicurist whose clients include Mariah Carey, Catherine Zeta-Jones, Gisele Bündchen, Heidi Klum, Penelope Cruz, and Salma Hayek.

Jennifer Leung: owner and founder of the Lavande Nail Spa in San Francisco.

Jessica Vartoughian: dubbed the First Lady of Nails by the *New York Times*, Vartoughian is Hollywood's leading natural nail–care specialist.

Jin Soon Choi: the owner of two Manhattan nail spas which regularly make *New York* magazine's Best of New York list, Choi's regular clients include Julianne Moore and Sarah Jessica Parker.

Marsha Bialo: Hollywood-based celebrity manicurist affiliated with OPI whose work has graced the hands of Kate Hudson, Beyonce, Renee Zellweger, Jessica Simpson, Gretchen Mol, Gwen Stefani, Eva Longoria, Teri Hatcher, and Alicia Keys.

Skyy Hadley: creator of the As "U" Wish Nail Spa in Hoboken, New Jersey, her clients include Faith Evans, Uma Thurman, Sean "Diddy" Combs, Liv Tyler, Mariska Hargitay, Alicia Keys, Kelly Rowland, and Chris Webber.

Wende Zomnir: creative director of Hard Candy Cosmetics and founder/creative director of Urban Decay Cosmetics.

Jim Miller: founder of California North, a West Coast skin-care line.

HAND-Y TIPS

The Buzz from the Beauty Editor

I have recently noticed a change in my hands. They are a little dryer, with more fine lines. Since I've always taken pride in my hands, this development has been pretty distressing. So when I leave the house, I replace my hand cream with sunscreen, and I keep pumps of lotion at every single sink in the house. I've made it a habit to smooth on some lotion after every handwashing.

Insider Information from the Beauty Bunch

Attack Aging

"Always wear sunblock on your hands to prevent signs of aging." Elisa Ferri

Aging Hands

"There are a few ways to help heal dry, chapped hands. First, try using a good hand cream that will nourish and heal the skin. Glycolic acid is helpful in exfoliating dry skin and reducing pigmentation spots due to age or sun. Second, try wearing gloves (two pairs—thin cotton gloves beneath the latex gloves to absorb any excess water) while cleaning or when hands are exposed to water. Third, make sure to wear wool or cashmere gloves during cold weather. Fourth, wear gloves outdoors while gardening as a protective barrier. It's really important to keep applying a hand cream several times a day, especially after your hands have been exposed to water." Giella

Hand Habit

"Do your entire skin-care routine on your hands as well, since they are one of the first places to show aging." Peter Thomas Roth

Hand Help

"Invest in salon treatments as well as at-home care when you have severe dryness of the hands or feet. Try paraffin treatments in the salon regularly until you see a major improvement. That can also be followed up at home with a soft exfoliator and thick hand and foot creams. If you live in a cold climate, please wear your winter gloves! That will help prevent the skin on your hands from getting chapped. Wear gloves when using cleaning products, even though it is more tempting to dig in there to do the cleaning without. Chemicals can really dry out your skin." Dee Pearn

Power of Paraffin

"Paraffin treatments will help to keep the hands and feet moist and soft." Jennifer Leung

Dry-Skin Defeaters

"Unfortunately, we all get older, which dries out our skin on our hands and feet. Excessive sun and harsh chemicals can increase the dryness factor in our skin as well. The key is moisture, moisture, and more moisture. Everyone should apply hand and body lotion after their morning shower, while still damp, and reapply hand lotion throughout the day. It is also important to apply your cuticle cream or oil in the morning. For baby-smooth skin, I strongly recommend applying your cuticle cream or oil as well as a rich hand and body lotion like our Hand & Body Emulsion on both hands and feet, and then wearing white gloves and white socks overnight so the cream will penetrate the skin. You will wake up soft and supple all over. If possible, you should do this at least three times a week." Jessica Vartoughian

Skin Soothers

"If you have really dry hands, use a shea-butter cream. L'Occitane makes a really good one. My client used it and said it was wonderful. In Fiore also makes a good one, and Kiehl's makes a good cuticle cream. This is for heavy duty use. In general, just use a regular hand cream, like Ahava, after you wash your hands." Jin Soon Choi

Hand Spa

"You can do a wonderful treatment at home. Take a little bit of sugar and a little bit of oil, any kind you have in the house, olive or vegetable or avocado; I like the richer oils. Mix it with some lemon juice to form a paste, and rub it on hands. The acidity in the lemon juice cleans. It's a great treatment. You can also do it on your feet. Another treatment is to grind up poppy seeds in a coffee grinder, add a little baking soda, half a cup of sugar, and water or oil. Rub it on legs and feet. Poppy seeds provide a little friction. It's exfoliating and stimulating for your skin." Marsha Bialo

MANICURE BASICS

The Buzz from the Beauty Editor

I'm obsessed with manicures, and I try to get one every single week. When my nails are sloppy, I actually feel dirty. A manicure appointment makes me feel fresh again. No matter how casual you are, beautiful nails make you look polished and pulled together.

Insider Information from the Beauty Bunch

Skyy's Secret

"My secret is to stop using water during a manicure. It brings moisture out of the hands and nails, and the nail horn needs to have eighteen-percent moisture in it. Instead, I use baggies with hot cream and essential oils. Let hands sit in the cream bag for ten seconds instead of water for five seconds. Faith Evans just came in for this." Skyy Hadley

The Long and Short of It

The ideal nail length is "about half an inch past the tip of your finger, or a quarter of an inch. I don't like super-long nails. But the length has more to do with trends or style or how the person wants to show themselves to the world. Nails are an accessory, like jewelry." Marsha Bialo

Pre-Polish

"The surface of the nail needs to be dry for the polish to last. I always clean the surface with Scrub Fresh from Creative Nail Design to remove the oils and residue from the manicure, letting the polish adhere to the nails." Skyy Hadley

Starworthy Manicure Tips

"When I developed my system, it was important to create simple and essential techniques to help grow and maintain nails for both the professional manicurist and the client. You should soak your nails before filing. If you file a dry nail, you separate the layers of keratin, which can cause peeling. If you soak the nail first, the nail expands and you will file the nail without causing any trauma or separation. It is important to apply all treatments and color, under and over the nail, while sealing the edges. This will encase the nail, seal in the moisture, and prevent breaking and chipping. You should also use eight to ten strokes when applying your polish. This will give a rich coverage and help the nails dry faster." Jessica Vartoughian

Manicure Maneuvers

"A great manicure is a whole package, from beginning to end. I'm very detail-oriented. I care for each step. I don't file the side of the nails too much, which ruins your nails. When the nails grow out, the sides won't grow out. Or it can produce a hangnail. I clean quickly and then go to the corner. And don't file too strongly. Do it softly. And I push back the cuticles really thoroughly." Jin Soon Choi

Flawless Filing

"The biggest mistake women make in filing their nails is using a seesaw motion. The trick is in the type of file. Use a low-grade file, like a diamond file, and file in one direction as much as possible. Then file downward at the nail tip to seal nail layers together and strengthen nails. Getting results is not about doing it hard; it's about doing as little as possible." Marsha Bialo

Pro Pointers

"Always make sure the nail plate is clean and dry before applying basecoat. Polish three strokes down and swipe across the tip so that the color will stay longer. Reapply topcoat the next day to help polish last. We apply our very own cuticle cream on clients to keep their cuticles moist and to keep them from peeling." Jennifer Leung

Polish Tips

"I like to load up the brush with polish, wipe off one side of the brush completely and start stroking the polish onto the middle of the nail with a light stroke. I go towards one side wall, start in the middle again and work my way to the other side wall. Putting too much pressure when you polish might cause the polish to streak. Stay away from the cuticle, but not too far where it looks like you have one-week growth!" Dee Pearn

Million-Dollar Manicure Tips

"The first thing you have to do, if you want to make your polish last long, is get rid of all the grease from your nail bed. Grease-free is very important. The nail polish won't stick there. Apply a basecoat, then apply two coats of nail polish, and dab some extra on the tip of your nail. Do the same thing with the top-coat; touch up the tip of your nail. Apply polish properly. First, don't touch the cuticle with the nail polish. Don't make too much of a gap right below the cuticle; you shouldn't see any bare nail, but don't touch. It's very important for me to make a smooth connection right below the cuticle. Sometimes, the line is not connected and that looks ugly. Follow your cuticle line, and keep it nicely connected. I also don't apply the polish in a straight line, especially when I do the sides of the nails. I see a lot of manicurists apply nail polish straight, but I apply polish in the curve of the side of your nails. I follow the curve in a circular motion, following the natural nail shape. And I use thin coats. I don't like thick coats. It depends on the color, but in general, I keep the coats thin." Jin Soon Choi

Warm Fuzzies

"I have noticed my clients comment on how warm and lovely my lotion feels when I start doing my hand and arm massage. They look for the lotion warmer. My secret? I dispense the cold lotion onto my hands, rub it in my hands for ten seconds to warm it up, and start applying. They love it!" Dee Pearn

The Jessica Manicure

"I have had the honor of training manicurists all over the world, and once they learn my system and techniques, they never go back to the way they did nails before. A great manicure should be therapeutic and pampering for the ultimate experience. Proper techniques for lasting wear are essential, [and so is] the correct basecoat treatment to solve any nail problem so nails can grow long, strong, and most importantly, healthy. [It should also include] a wonderful hand massage with a rich, non-oily cream or lotion. We include a hot thermal mitten treatment in the Jessica Manicure." Jessica Vartoughian

Clean Sweep

"Whether nails are short or long, the important thing is to keep them clean, with no chipped polish. There's a wonderful product you can use to clean nails; it's a soap called Lava. It's a very good soap for getting rid of heavy-duty dirty hands, but it's very drying, so it's important to use lotions. That is the key. Keep your feet and your hands clean." Marsha Bialo

Step-by-Step Manicure

"A great manicure should start with clean hands. Removing the old polish is then followed by a shaping of the nails. I always ask the client what it is that they are looking for, and together we come up with a plan. A cuticle product should be applied to loose, dead skin that is stuck on the nail plate. Many nail techs have gotten away from using the soaking bowl; either they are cutting corners for time or maybe they are using products that don't involve the use of a warm, sudsy finger bath. I guess I am old school because I still believe that is the way to go. It helps clean out under the nails and it helps you see the little pieces of nail that did not quite get filed off, so you can bevel them off now. After the cuticles are pushed back and cleaned up, I like to buff the nails with oil and a soft buffing file to help smooth out the ridges and clean up any stains on the nail plate. What the client finds the best about the manicure, besides a great polish job, is the hand and arm massage. Give a good one, and they will be happy. Give a great one, and they will want to come back for more! It is very important that the lotions and oils are removed off of the nail plate after the massage and before polish application to prevent polish from peeling. Wipe nails with sanitizer and polish remover before polishing with basecoat, two coats of color, and a topcoat. After waiting a few minutes, I sometimes like to apply drying drops. This is an oil-based solution that is dropped on the nails to help speed up the drying time as well as condition the cuticles. This works great when we are working on the set and are pressed for time. During photo shoots, I like to apply a fast-drying topcoat. We need the polish dry ASAP and will probably be changing it several times throughout the day. In the salon, I like to apply a thicker topcoat, one that will be long-lasting for the week." Dee Pearn

Application Advice

"Always make sure the nail is clean and dry. Don't put lotion on before you polish. Do it after your hands are dry later on. Lotion absorbs into crevices of nails and causes polish to chip. Don't put polish too close to the cuticle because oils in the cuticles cause polish to chip. Fan out the brush to get close to the cuticle. Wait a few seconds before fixing mistakes, because it's easier to remove polish if it's a little dry." Marsha Bialo

No Pain, All Gain

"Always remember: a manicure should not hurt! It should be a pleasant experience. I have had so many clients say, 'Wow! That didn't even hurt! You are so gentle!' I have even heard, 'Wow! I didn't even bleed this time!' Are you kidding me? They just figured that's what you have to go through for beauty." Dee Pearn

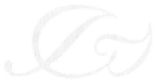

SHAPE TALK

The Buzz from the Beauty Editor
In my opinion, the most modern shape for nails is short and slightly squared off. Long nails are harsh, out of style, and hygienically challenged. Shorter nails look fresh, clean, and sophisticated, and they can pull off any polish color you choose.

Insider Information from the Beauty Bunch

Shape Up

"No nail shape is wrong. You just have to find the right thing that works for you. A lot of women like to go sharp in corners, but if you take off the corner or file too much on the sides of your nail, they generally won't grow out as well. For most people, their nails grow out better if the sides are straight, but for some people, their nails won't grow like that. The popular shape right now is a rounded-off square, but if your body cannot handle an oval or square nail, then that doesn't work for you." Marsha Bialo

Ship Shape

"Nail shape should be determined by your cuticle. For oval-shaped cuticles, oval-shaped nails look best, and for square-shaped cuticles, square-shaped nails look best. For those with an in-between shape, I suggest a square shape with rounded edges. Because so many women are so busy these days, they don't have as much time to take care of those gorgeous nails and are keeping them simple and short. This way, women have the ability to work freely with their hands and still looked groomed and polished without having to keep up with it as frequently. The hottest trend among celebrities is the round nail shape, kept short with a neutral polish." Jessica Vartoughian

Chic Shape

"[Today, women are] not wearing their nails too long. Now, people wear them short, right above the fingertips. Not round or square, more of a natural square. Kristin Davis has that shape and length." Jin Soon Choi

Shaping Up

"The ideal nail shape and length in my opinion is the square-oval, or 'squoval.' It is flat on the top, but rounded on the corners. I find that the majority of my in-salon clientele ask for that the most. It seems to give them that modern look without the corners catching and breaking off. The length that is very popular is just a little bit of nail past the finger tip. Very clean and classy. Most of my celebrity clients, like Catherine-Zeta Jones and Penelope Cruz, prefer the same. Beyonce, on the other hand, had me file hers more oval and we kept them a little bit longer. They were naturally beautiful and suited her nail beds." Dee Pearn

Preferred Shape

"Most of our clients prefer a relatively short length, squared at the tips but [with] rounded corners." Jennifer Leung

MANICURE MISTAKES

The Buzz from the Beauty Editor

One of the biggest mistakes, according to the pros, is buying nail-care products and not using them. If you want your manicure to last, you have to apply a topcoat every couple of days. If you want your cuticles to be healthy, you have to apply cuticle oil or cream on a regular basis. Don't just buy those nail products. Use them!

Insider Information from the Beauty Bunch

Peelin' Polish

"Never peel off your polish when you feel like taking it off! That could damage your own nail plate as you peel off some of your nail along with the polish! Always use polish remover." Dee Pearn

Color Over Care

"At home, the biggest mistake is that women don't use their products. They buy them and let them sit there. They have to really use the products. That's why hands and nails are dry. Women don't actually push back the cuticle at home properly. Cuticle has a shape too. When you push it back nicely, you can see a nice rounded shape. When your cuticle is clean, it's easier to apply polish and it looks much better. Women don't use cuticle oil or cream on their nail beds, but your nail beds need moisture too. They focus more on color than on care." Jin Soon Choi

Nail No-No's

"Not taking the advice of your nail tech [is a mistake]! Sometimes clients are advised to use an at-home nail treatment in between visits. It is easier said than done! It doesn't work as good sitting on the shelf! Another mistake would be picking at your dry cuticles instead of moisturizing them often with creams or oils." Dee Pearn

Manicure Spoilers

"For a pedicure, putting closed-toe shoes on too early, before the polish is dry, is a big mistake. For a manicure: digging in your purse right after your polish is put on. Or talking on the phone during polish application. Hair gets caught in the polish, nails are bumped against the phone, and it's just a nightmare to fix." Dee Pearn

CUTICLE CUES

The Buzz from the Beauty Editor

Just in case you are still wondering, cutting cuticles is a definite no-no. The best manicurists know that trimming this delicate area destroys their shape, leaves them raggedy, and opens you up to infection.

Insider Information from the Beauty Bunch

Cuticle Dream

"Cuticles will only do well if they're moisturized and protected. Neosporin is a wonderful antibacterial that heals cuticles, but if they are always splitting or dry, go to a dermatologist or a podiatrist to find out how to heal the skin so your nails will grow." Marsha Bialo

Cuticle Cutting?

"Cuticles should not be cut, if you can help it. Cuticles are there for a reason. If we start cutting away at the cuticles, then we open up the risk of getting an inflamed cuticle wall, getting an infection in the matrix area, or having overgrowth caused by overcutting where the body naturally starts reproducing more cuticle to repair the damage. Some manicurists cut and pull pieces off the cuticle which is not only damaging, but then the cuticle grows back ragged and always wants to peel. I only cut a cuticle if it is extremely overgrown or if there is a hangnail, or a piece of damaged cuticle from the past is just waving up in the air and is an eyesore!" Dee Pearn

Cuticle Caution

The biggest mistake you can make? "Cutting cuticles. I do not believe in cutting away all the cuticles, preferring to gently nip away hangnails and dry loose skin surrounding the nail plate only." Jennifer Leung

Trimming Cuticles

Should cuticles be cut? "No, no, no, no, no, no. When a nail tech cuts a cuticle, they need to know how to leave the main cuticle, because when they cut the main cuticle, that's a problem. Sometimes there is an exception; sometimes you have to trim. When you push back the cuticle thoroughly, you'll see the part of the cuticle that looks like its hanging or raggedy. Don't touch the main line. It tears off. Some people have no definition of the main cuticle. Some manicurists think cutting it all off will look good, but a few days later the cuticle comes back and looks awful. Why bother to get a manicure? Push back cuticles at home and apply cuticle oil and cream." Jin Soon Choi

Quick Fix

"If you don't have cuticle remover, take toothpaste, the white kind not the gel kind, and put it around the cuticles of the hands or feet. Then take a toothbrush and scrub your toenails and hands, and rub the toothpaste on your nails. It's a wonderful way to clean." Marsha Bialo

Cuticle Care

"Applying cuticle oil daily is so important. It helps eliminate the dryness, therefore stopping the urge to pick and peel." Dee Pearn

Soothing Soak

Best way to care for cuticles? "Moisture, moisture, moisture. Use a cuticle cream that is made from natural plant oils and vitamin E, or you can mix your own cuticle treatment by blending one teaspoon jojoba oil and vitamin-E oil with a half teaspoon of honey. Soak your nails for ten minutes and apply lotion to your hands. Do this routine twice a week." Jennifer Leung

COLOR CUES

The Buzz from the Beauty Editor

One of my favorite polish shades is a pinkish-white neutral, and I am constantly on the prowl for new versions of this color. Some are too sheer; others, too opaque. Many are too pink, and a few, too white. Color selection can be tricky. That's why, when you find a color you love, you should make a note of the name. Keep a bottle at home for between-manicure touch-ups.

Insider Information from the Beauty Bunch

Flight of Fancy

"When you travel, wear a sparkly sheer color—chips aren't as noticeable when your nails get banged around a lot from handling luggage." Wende Zomnir

Pick a Color

"Colors should be chosen by personal choice. After that, a little direction from the nail tech is always good to help decide if it blends into your skintone too much, or if the color is just not doing anything for you and there is another one that's better. The best way to find out is to just put the bottle of polish against your skin and see, even when picking a neutral color. Depending on your skintone, some neutral colors may look too yellow or too bright pink. Always ask the nail tech to do a test on your fingernail to get a better look. If they roll their eyes at you, then roll right out of there! It's time to go elsewhere, where you can freely figure out what color is best for you." Dee Pearn

Skintone Tips

"Bright and sparkly color complements tanned skin and is always good for summer. Pastels are great for fair skin. It is always safe to choose a flattering neutral." Jennifer Leung

French Feat

"Right now, French is more popular on toes in a thin line, but not on fingers. The French pedicure is more popular. Don't do thick lines for a French manicure. It's cheap-looking. Make sure the white line is not too thick. And you don't always have to do a classic French manicure. You can create your own colors, or do a reverse French, which is white with a pink line." Jin Soon Choi

Neutral Cues

"Sheer tones of pink or beige are a great neutral look. What also looks great, especially for the summer, is a light but opaque pink, almost like a bubble-gum pink, but lighter. That was the color chosen by Mariah Carey when we worked together last. Lately, going even more natural than ever is in. I discovered this while working with Mario Testino just recently. His direction to me was to create a look that was natural for Carolyn Murphy, but he did not want to see any color at all, and no shine, but it had to look like she had her nails done. I brainstormed, and after I did her manicure, I applied two coats of a matte-finish basecoat. The look was exactly what he was looking for. It looked awesome, and I thank him for the challenge. After that, I fell in love with that look and use it often on both male and female clients." Dee Pearn

Shade Shopping

"Like makeup, you should choose shades that complement your skintone. Since your skin color may change slightly from season to season, I suggest working with colors that fit for your skintone for each season. For fair skin, berry-reds work best. Deeper burgundies are more flattering for those with a medium skintone. Olive complexions look best with a goldish tone or a dark red or purple. For those with dark skin, I suggest brighter pinks and reds." Jessica Vartoughian

French Fan?

"I am not a big fan of French manicures or pedicures but that doesn't mean I am against them. Having off-white color on the tip area will certainly make them look fresher." Jennifer Leung

Classic Colors

"I love sheers. That's my thing. My favorite for hands is natural, and for toes, red. That is the most flattering, classic combination that can't go wrong. You don't have to follow trends. This will always be in style." Jin Soon Choi

Sheer and Clear

"I like to put sheer on fingernails; however, if there is a little flaw in the nail plate, it is always nice to cover that up first with an opaque color in the same family followed by a sheer one. It is always fun to change it up a bit with a little sparkle now and then." Dee Pearn

Winning Colors

"[I like] Miso Happy With This Color by OPI for fingers and Organdy by Chanel or Pansy by Essie for toes." Jennifer Leung

Navigating Neutrals

"A flattering neutral looks beautiful with a tan or a medium skintone, but doesn't look as good on someone who has fair skin. When the colors of the skin and nails blend, it looks as if you have no nails." Jessica Vartoughian

Fabulous French

"I think the French manicure for hands and feet is always very classy. It's Ashanti's choice every time we work together. In modern times, a soft French is very appealing. Soft French is when the white is a few shades lighter than the very opaque white, and then you finish it off with a very sheer pink or beige.

Having your nails done in French and your toes done in a solid color is also very acceptable. I love seeing a soft French on the hands and a fun bright color on the toes. Classy hands with flirty toes. The perfect blend. There is a misconception that you need to have long nails for a French manicure. Absolutely not! It can be done on nails that have no free edge at all. That's the beauty of the French. Short French is classy. Sometimes, clients have one nail that is shorter than the rest. Instead of making it longer with an artificial nail, just put a white free edge on that broken nail and suddenly, the eye is tricked into thinking the nail has a free edge!" Dee Pearn

Sheer Beauty
"I love sheer colors, but for some reason, nail polish with sparkle seems to last longer." Jennifer Leung

French Choices
"I am very partial to a classic French manicure for nails. We offer a wide array of neutral shades in pinks, beiges, lavenders, and different textured whites so that you can customize the perfect color combination for your French manicure. It also gives you the option to change your look with each manicure." Jessica Vartoughian

Mix It Up
"You ultimately have to know your color chart, but orange-pinks and cream colors seem to go with everyone. You want to try to stay away from cream colors with a yellow base. They can make nails look dingy. I tend to like opaques or opaques with a little frost in them. Don't be afraid to mix colors. I mix them all the time. If you find a color that's too yellow, add some white. But be sure to mix colors within the same brand; don't mix different brands. They won't blend and the polish bottle will explode." Marsha Bialo

Contrasting Colors
"I always check the skintone. I don't match their skintone. I go more for contrast. It's more flattering. Some people have pink-toned skin and they use a pink color, which is not really good. Use a dark color pink, not a sheer color, for contrast. If they want to go natural, I go for a mix of natural white with natural pink. Contrast with your skintone is really good. Don't match your skintone if you use a dark color. For example, with olive or yellow skintones, don't go beige. Use a pinkish or whitish or combination. Olive has good tones, so olive skin can wear most colors. Avoid beige and you'll be fine." Jin Soon Choi

Toe Shades
"Toes should be where your creativity comes out and you can be more daring. Bright, fun shades in pinks and reds, or even a tint of gold for the summer, which is my all-time favorite. They make your toes stand out in those sexy sandals. A dark red is great for winter and even a little festive for the holidays." Jessica Vartoughian

MANICURE MAINTENANCE

The Buzz from the Beauty Editor
I am really hard on my nails, and I'm also a notorious klutz, so I am constantly on the search for products and techniques designed to make my manicure last the week. I always wear gloves when I wash dishes, even if it's a single glass, and sometimes, I even wear plastic gloves when cooking. Protecting your manicure is one way to make it last; the other

way is to get a great manicure to begin with. Here, the pros show you how to make that happen.

Insider Information from the Beauty Bunch

Chip Prevention

"After you get a manicure, you should purchase the same color nail polish and a bottle of Nailtiques. There are four types of Nailtiques, so ask your manicurist which is better for you. Number 2 is the most common. Every morning, apply a coat of polish to the tips of your nails, and then apply one coat of Nailtiques. It is fast-drying, so you should not have any smudges. This will take care of your nail chipping, and your nails will be stronger, too." Giella

Marathon Manicure

"If you want your manicure to last seven to eight days, without a chip, I've got a special system for that. You start with a coat of Trind Moisturizing Nail Balsam, then a coat of Nailtiques No. 2, then Zoya polish, then Nailtiques No. 2 again. I guarantee your manicure will last. If you can't find Trind, use a basecoat instead." Skyy Hadley

Lasting Color

"Make sure to get rid of any excess oil on the nail bed before applying basecoat. Choose a basecoat that bonds the color, such as Bonder from Orly. Topcoat is also very important to keep the polish from chipping—reapply topcoat for three days after your manicure." Jennifer Leung

Staying Power

"If you are really hard on your hands, you want to polish them with a light color so that if it chips, it won't show. Keep the color with you. Or skip polish and get them lightly buffed. Wear gloves. Don't use your hands as tools to pick your teeth." Marsha Bialo

Keeping Up Appearances

"I always advise clients to apply a thin clear coat in two days, then again in two more days. That way it seals in the color and the wear and tear you do with your hands rubs off the clear, not the color. To prolong a pedicure, I suggest putting lotion on your feet daily, especially after having a pedicure where the dryness is removed, so the lotion can absorb into the skin and keep your feet from feeling rough. I would also apply a thick clear coat on them once a week. If you go to the beach daily, after taking a shower after the beach, apply a thin clear coat on the toenails, which are dulled by the sand. Wear slippers! It makes a big difference! Walking on the floor, whether carpet or hardwood or tile, is very drying to your feet. Slip those fuzzy slippers on and keep your feet soft." Dee Pearn

Staying Power

"To properly maintain a manicure for long-lasting wear, you should apply your topcoat the day after your treatment and then apply another coat of color and topcoat every three to four days thereafter until your next manicure. Cuticle oil or cream should be massaged into cuticles every day." Jessica Vartoughian

Frequent Visits

"Get a manicure once a week, and a pedicure twice a month. To maintain a manicure, apply topcoat the next day after your manicure and reapply for the next two days. Wear gloves when you do dishes or garden." Jennifer Leung

No-Chip Nails

"Do not be thrifty when using a basecoat and a topcoat. That will help prolong your initial manicure.

After that, it is up to you and how hard you are on your nails in your everyday activity. Wear gloves when gardening and washing the dishes. Put cuticle oil on often. Wear hand creams." Dee Pearn

Regular Visits
"For best results, a woman should get a manicure every ten days and a pedicure every three to four weeks." Jessica Vartoughian

Salon Schedule
"Get a manicure once a week, and a pedicure every two to three weeks." Jin Soon Choi

Protect Your Polish
"Keep the lid on tight and store nail polish in a cool dark place out of sunlight. Polish will last if it is a full bottle. Once the polish is half empty, the air inside will cause the polish to dry in the bottle. Many nail techs like to thin it out with polish thinners. I, personally, would not do that. I have found that it changes the consistency of the polish, where it streaks going on, or if it does go on well, it takes *forever* to dry. In some cases, it never really does. I can't afford to take that risk. I just start a fresh bottle when I feel like my polish is not workable anymore." Dee Pearn

NAIL HEALTH

The Buzz from the Beauty Editor
Beautiful nails are by definition healthy, and healthy nails are strong yet flexible. If your nails are naturally healthy, read on for ways to keep them that way, and if you suffer from split, weak, peeling nails, you'll find strategies to get your nails into their best shape ever.

Insider Information from the Beauty Bunch

Doctor's Orders
With nail strengtheners, "it's hit-or-miss with everyone. You have to experiment, because everyone's body chemistry is different. The best thing to do is go to your dermatologist, who has lotions or creams that can help nails. Any kind of lotion with ammonium lactate in it can help nails grow." Marsha Bialo

Flexible Fingertips
"If nails are too hard, they break, which is why you want them flexible. That's why I prefer a nail strengthener to a nail hardener, which makes them too strong. If you want flexibility to your nails, and you can't afford to come in every week for a manicure, I suggest keeping hands out of water, using an AHA product, and using a cream instead of a lotion. Use a scrub of sugar, oatmeal, and Solar Oil. It's a mask and a scrub in one, and it brightens up the skin. You don't need to leave it on. Just scrub and rinse. Another key to that youthful look is paraffin, but keep it on for less than five minutes. You don't need anything to sit. Leave it too long and you'll dry it out. Too much of anything is wrong. Less is best." Skyy Hadley

Weak-Nail Rx
"Weak, splitting nails should be shortened until they get on the right track only because the longer they are with splits in them, the more susceptible they are to snagging on clothing and such, causing them to

tear off. There are many products out on the market that are geared specifically to splitting nails. They need to be used as directed. The key to that is: do not overuse! Once you see the results you are looking for, stop using that formula and switch to something else. Otherwise, you may overuse it which will cause reverse effects." Dee Pearn

Save Splitting Nails

"Use a nail strengthener that contains protein and calcium. If that does not work, try a silk wrap." Jennifer Leung

Care and Repair

"No one wants a hand with only four fingernails. If you don't take care of splitting nails, they may completely break off. You can save them with extra protection during the initial growth phase. We have a product called Life Jacket that is formulated with natural fibers that help cushion the nail and reinforce the split while the nail grows out. It is applied horizontally and vertically to create a weave. Since it has natural fibers, we recommend our Flawless Ridge Filler be applied after the Life Jacket to create a smooth surface for the application of color." Jessica Vartoughian

Feed Your Nails

"Take vitamins. Prenatal vitamins make your nails strong. How they work I don't know, but it is amazing. I've seen many, many pregnant women whose hair and nails get so much stronger after taking the vitamins. You can also take Omega-3 or eat a lot of fish. Find a proper nail strengthener; the right one depends on the person. Moisturize your nail bed. Put a lot of oil and cream on your nails. Even strong nails can become brittle and dry because there's not enough moisture. Your nails need moisture as much as your face." Jin Soon Choi

Weak-Nail Wonder

"If you have splitting, chipped nails, and you cut your nail, you close the seam. The nail is composed of layers, and when they aren't sealed, they tend to split. After you cut them, file the nail in one direction, and then go on top of your nail and file downward to close the seam. Don't be afraid to file the top of your nail. Heat caused by friction separates the nail tissue, which prevents it from growing. Ultimately you don't want to take the corners off your nail, because it's the foundation for your nails to grow. You [don't want to] take away that foundation." Marsha Bialo

Fungus Culprits

"It is a myth that you can only get fungus if you wear artificial nails. You can have natural nails and poke yourself with something under the nail, damaging the tissue and causing an infection that, if not looked after, can turn into a mold or fungus. A hairdresser can get hair splinters under their fingernails or toenails." Dee Pearn

Inside Out

"Drink water. It's vital to nail health." Marsha Bialo

Strengthener Strategy

"If you feel a burning sensation when using a nail strengthener, it means you are putting it on the skin. It should not touch the skin or the cuticle area. Put it on carefully. We tend to get sloppy because it is clear and no one will see the mistakes." Dee Pearn

Fungus Fixers

"Why do frequent travelers, like athletes or business people, get fungus on their feet? I don't believe the housekeepers in hotels clean the showers very well. Carry Lysol or bleach with you when you travel and use it to rinse down the shower or tub. Foot fungus on avid travelers is primarily caused by dirty showers. If you're on a trip and your feet are itching you, pee on your feet to kill the fungus. There's a component of urine, the acidity, that can kill athlete's foot or fungus until you can get to a doctor. Madonna mentioned this tip once. A combination of bleach and water on a cotton swab can also kill fungus." Marsha Bialo

TIMELESS TOOLS

The Buzz from the Beauty Editor

Manicure tools seem innocent enough, but they can harbor a variety of diseases and infections. That's why it's so important to make sure that your salon properly sterilizes all of its tools. Better yet, take your own set of implements, and you'll never have to worry.

Insider Information from the Beauty Bunch

Top Tools

"The first tool you need for a great manicure is a bright light. You need to see the work you do as brightly as you can. Dim lighting helps [the manicurist] get away with more, but once the client goes outside and sees polish slapped all over the place, don't be surprised if you hear tire tracks screeching out of there and never coming back! Other than the lighting, there are a few other good tools I find necessary: a very gentle and sturdy cuticle pusher, one that won't damage the nail plate or tear the cuticle.

Also, a corrector pen. I dip it in polish remover and clean up any mistakes made fast and easy without mess. The tip of the corrector pen is easily replaced between clients for sanitary reasons. Another tool I could not live without is my custom-cut paint brush. I use it to clean off the nail surface of creams and oils before polishing the nail. By doing it this way, instead of using a cotton ball, it is cleaner and easier than trying to get all the lint off the nail from the cotton before polishing." Dee Pearn

Rank and File

"A file and a good base and topcoat [are indispensable]. Soft Touch [makes] the best file." Jennifer Leung

Fine Files

"Get a nice, proper file. Wash it after you use it. Diamond nail files are good to have. Try to find a file with a very fine grain. A strong grain will harm your nails. If you don't have time, you can quickly file and put polish on. A cuticle pusher is also important." Jin Soon Choi

True Grit

"Look for a nail file with a low grit, like one with a 100–180 grit factor, which is relatively smooth or fine. Feel the file. If it's really harsh or has too much grit, don't use it. I also like OPI PusherGuard Sensitive Cuticle Pusher and Blue Cross Cuticle Remover." Marsha Bialo

Favorite File

"I love a file that is long-lasting and easily disinfected. Two of my very favorites are the Tammy Taylor Natural Nail Shaper and the Nail Tek Crystal Nail File. I love them both." Dee Pearn

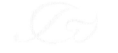

SALON SENSE

The Buzz from the Beauty Editor

A salon's hygiene practices are even more important than the quality of its manicures. Preliminary hygiene concerns can be addressed with a quick look around the salon. Beyond that, there are a few key things to look for, and our experts show you what they are.

Insider Information from the Beauty Bunch

Speak Up

"Ask questions! Are there any unmarked bottles on the table and you have no idea what is being applied on you? A confident tech should have no problems answering your questions or concerns." Dee Pearn

Attitude Counts

"A good manicure is a full package. What's the attitude of the nail tech? Is there attention to detail? How does the tech file? Does it touch the skin? Because that is annoying. How do they do all the different steps? If you know manicures, you see it right away." Jin Soon Choi

Tech Talk

"Choose a skilled technician who understands your needs. If there is a bad smell in a nail salon, you want to walk away. Also, check to make sure the spa chair is clean and if the salon has a sanitation log." Jennifer Leung

Salon Assessment

"No one wants a Paula Abdul episode [Abdul nearly lost a thumb to an infection after a visit to an unsanitary nail salon in April 2004], and yet it's fairly easy to detect! A clean salon environment is so important; your nails extend underneath your skin.* First, you can look at a manicurist's table, and if her table is messy and disorganized, this should be a red flag. If her bottles are dirty and her implements are not soaking in disinfectant, I would strongly reevaluate getting my nails done at the salon. A good salon will have all bottles and disinfectants clearly labeled, and all implements should be immersed in Barbicide or alcohol and properly sanitized before beginning any treatment." Jessica Vartoughian

Salon Spy

"Sit and watch and see what they're doing; you really don't know until you watch. If they are using one of those whirlpool machines, are they rinsing it out and cleaning it? Are their tools in sanitary bags or in an Autoclave [a hospital-grade machine that is the most powerful way to sterilize], or do they use new tools on each client? How clean is the area where you're sitting? How clean are the bathrooms? Are they listening to what you have to say or do they want you in and out? If they are taking the time to listen to what you want, then they care about you." Marsha Bialo

Hygiene Check

"As a concerned client, there are things you should look for. If you are waiting for your manicure and

---

* Editor's Note: Since your nails extend underneath your skin, they actually go into your body. They are not just external. Therefore, a nail infection can cause damage that is more far-reaching than just the surface of the nail. It can get into the bloodstream.

you can see your nail tech finishing up with the client before you, watch her clean her station. Did she remove the towel off the table and replace it with a clean fresh one? Did she spray and wipe the table with disinfectant before doing so? What did she do with the files? Did she pull out fresh, clean files for you or is she using dirty files she just used on the last five people before you? Are her implements fully submerged in a disinfectant covered by a lid? Does she have a hot lotion warmer on her table without a lid, collecting dust and bacteria? Does she use the same orangewood stick for several clients? Did your nail tech drop an implement on the floor, pick it up, and continue working on you without disinfecting it first? When it comes to using a paraffin bath, is the paraffin being applied on you or are you being dipped into it, which can cause cross-contamination from client to client? Are the pedicure baths being properly cleaned between clients? If there are nail dryers there, are the dryers being disinfected after the use of *each* client? Or are you being escorted over to the nail dryer and putting your hands on top of someone else's leftover oil slick? Finally, if the nail tech blows on your finger to clear the dust, instead of using a manicure brush, do not sit with her again! She is blowing bacteria onto your finger and towards your face!" Dee Pearn

Hygiene Counts

"Ask about the salon's hygiene practices. Or bring your own tools. After the tools are sterilized, we put them in individual packages for that client. Check the file. Are they using a blue liquid [Barbicide], or an autoclave?" Jin Soon Choi

Curiosity Counts

"Being a good nail tech means keeping your ears open and being willing to learn new ideas from coworkers as well as clients. I meet all kinds of women and men that travel the world, and I just absorb their knowledge of what they have had done out there. I don't act insulted that they are giving me advice. I take it and thank them. This summer a client brought me a special buffing cream from Japan to shine up his nails with. I never would have known about it. Another client gave me the idea of using a toothpick to clean up polish that has ran into the side of the big toes, where the skin grows close up against the nail. These ideas are priceless." Dee Pearn

Appointment Etiquette

"Please come on time for your appointment! You are only cheating yourself if you don't. Why? What happens is the nail tech has two choices to make. Reschedule you or rush through the appointment. Chances are the tech does not want to lose money on that spot scheduled just for you, so she will take you and rush through your service. Rescheduling will only leave the client feeling upset and cheated. So please come on time! When booking an appointment, the biggest mistake I see is a client booking for a service that requires less time than what they really want. Like they book for a manicure, but they really want a manicure and five repairs, or a fill, or whatever. If you go to a tech that is busy back to back, chances of her being able to squeeze extra services in there are slim. Some clients do it on purpose, knowing that once they sit down, they won't be refused; others just don't know there is a difference. Explaining what it is exactly that you need on the phone when booking that appointment is important." Dee Pearn

Standing Appointments

"When wanting to have someone else care for your nails on a regular basis, it is common to get a manicure once a week and a pedicure once a month. There are others that come into the salon for a manicure only when their nails are very uneven and their cuticles need some care, and there are people who have a pedicure more often than just once a month." Dee Pearn

FAKE AND FABULOUS

The Buzz from the Beauty Editor
I'm not a fan of artificial nails; I prefer a more natural look. But if you want to wear your nails longer, and they simply refuse to grow, they can open up your options.

Insider Information from the Beauty Bunch

Artificial-Nail Intelligence
"There are many [artificial nail] products out there to choose from, and different nail techs apply them in their own way. It's hard to say which is the best. It all has to do with the individual. Sometimes a client is told bad things by a nail tech about a certain type of nail enhancement and she talks up another. Usually it is because they don't offer the one they are speaking badly about! Keep that in mind. What is best for you depends on how well you take to the different nail enhancements—acrylic, gel, fiberglass, silk—and how skilled the nail tech is at applying them. I hear clients tell me one type of nail enhancement is thinner than the other. Not necessarily true! It's all in the application! Scared clients tell me they have heard that nail enhancements damage your nails. I always tell them that yes, nail enhancements can be damag-

ing if the nail tech is drilling or filing by hand very roughly deep into the nail plate or too close to the cuticle, causing permanent damage, or if they rip off your nail enhancements instead of soaking them off. There are many ways to cause damage, but it doesn't have to be that way. I like to use Tammy Taylor acrylics. I love the fact that I can make them as thin or thick as needed. I don't use a drill on the nail plate, and I do soak them off when it's time, so there is no damage. The nail is just as weak or strong as it was before. It may feel a bit weak because we get used to having a shell protect our nail plate for so long, but by applying some nail strengthener the nails feel as good as new!" Dee Pearn

FANTASTIC FEET

The Buzz from the Beauty Editor
Living in Florida, a pedicure is a year-round essential. I think it's fun to be adventurous with pedicure polish, and I go a little crazy with the colors: corals, bright pinks, bold reds, even white.

Insider Information from the Beauty Bunch

Fancy Feet
"First of all, do not cut calluses with a razor! What is smooth now from the razor will be a big, ugly callous later! What works well is filing the callus dry with a foot file without soaking it first. It's a great way to remove all the dead dry skin. After that, apply

a thick foot lotion daily until feet are smooth again. Use the foot file only when dryness develops again. A word of advice if you go to the beach daily: the sand does a number on your feet, causing extreme dryness and dulling the toenail polish. Switch to sneakers. Protect those pedicured feet!" Dee Pearn

Soapy Soles

"When you take a shower or a bath, your feet naturally pick up all the soap deposits. The ring on your tub happens to your feet, too. They collect soap deposits and bacteria. That's not all cuticle that comes off—it's also soap and sweat deposits. Cut toenails straight across from corner to corner and clean around the cuticle." Marsha Bialo

Foot Fix

"Serious foot problems can only be treated by a podiatrist; however, wearing well-designed, comfortable shoes will certainly help to minimize the chance of having corns and bunions." Jennifer Leung

Shower Smoother

"Everyone should keep a pumice stone or foot file in their shower and apply an exfoliator like our ZenSpa Purifying Scrub daily. This will keep feet smooth and soft." Jessica Vartoughian

Odor Eraser

"For foot odor, soak feet in a tub of tea. The tannins in tea help foot odor." Marsha Bialo

Sole Savers

"First of all, I try to do it the natural way first, rather than using products. I recommend using a pumice stone during every single shower, and then using a non-greasy foot cream in the summer; in the winter, it can be heavier. And wear comfortable shoes. If you have a really bad callous, Elizabeth Arden Nail Care just launched a callous treatment. You put it on the callous and leave it for a while and then use a pumice stone." Jin Soon Choi

Baby-Bottom Soft

"Everyone has hard calluses on their feet. I have the best secret for getting rid of that. A&D Baby Ointment on your feet can get rid of calluses. It's only about five dollars, and the tube will last a year and a half. I heard it from a podiatrist and it's terrific. You mix some into your favorite lotion, whichever lotion you like. Keep it in a jar in the refrigerator so it doesn't melt." Marsha Bialo

Blister Beater

"In a pinch, if you are out on the street and you are starting to develop a blister, grab some Chapstick or lip gloss and put it on your blister area. Oil works well, too. If you are at a restaurant, dab a little olive oil on there when no one is looking!" Dee Pearn

Stiletto Helper

"Try liquid bandage on blisters." Jin Soon Choi

File Fetish

"The reason your feet get calloused is that your body loses moisture and the skin dries out. Friction—from walking and shoes and weather and showering—starts to diminish the elasticity in your feet. The Flowery Red Swedish Clover Foot File is the best [foot file] out there, ever. It really seems to work. The right way to buff feet is to make sure that they are damp; don't do it when they're dry. Get rid of callouses gently; don't use anything too abrasive. Keep feet as clean and moisturized as possible." Marsha Bialo

Foot Aid

Pedicures cannot be counted on to treat serious foot problems, like bunions or corns. "I don't like to use the word 'treat.' We are not doctors, and a lot of the time a client expects that from us. We are licensed to do pedicures, which can help soothe feet with bunions and corns. Using a foot file will, of course, improve the look of a foot with calluses on top of bunions. Any serious foot problems should be referred to a physician. Sometimes we get corns and bunions from the shoes we wear. Other times it is hereditary. I always refer those questions to a podiatrist." Dee Pearn

The Callous Question

"Use a callous-eliminator [cream] that breaks down callouses in about five minutes; follow by a paraffin treatment once a week." Jennifer Leung

Callous Cause

"You get [callouses and bunions] from your shoes, or from the way you walk. If you want to avoid them, you need comfortable shoes." Jin Soon Choi

Missing Nail Rescue

"Many times, I come across people who do not want polish on their toes because they broke a chunk of nail off the big toe and they are waiting for it to grow back. Why wait? Start enjoying life now and get a sculpted acrylic two-tone temporary toenail put on! It looks totally natural, and you don't have to be shy about open-toe shoes while your real nail grows out. This technique really came in handy on a recent shoot I did for a Gillette razor ad. The model was so happy to have a normal-looking toe, she almost cried. She called it her 'extreme makeover toe.'" Dee Pearn

The Petroleum Problem

"Petroleum jelly comforts and protects against weather damage, but it doesn't absorb. It doesn't resolve the problem. Find a product that heals or fixes." Marsha Bialo

Super Scrubber

"A scrub, like California North Gelskin Scrub, can be used to slough away dead skin cells on hands and feet." Jim Miller

Ingrown Alert

"If you have ingrown toenails, and you can't get to a salon, take scissors or a cuticle nipper and cut a V-shape into the tip of your big toenail. Make the V in the center of your toenail. It psyches out the nail. It thinks something is wrong and it starts growing. This isn't going to produce the best result, though. Ultimately, you do need someone to take care of them. There's a tool that I love by Tweezerman called the Ingrown Toenail File, but that's for a professional. The worst thing you can do is to try to fix it yourself." Marsha Bialo

THE PRODUCT FILES

Hand Treatments

The Buzz from the Beauty Editor

I've had plenty of experience with hand treatments. I love pampering my hands; some might say I'm a little obsessed. I've tried virtually everything on the market. These are the ones I come back to. Hand scrubs are a boon for hands, but they're hard on a manicure. That's why I use a scrub the night before my manicure appointment. Since I get weekly manicures, this system ensures that I am also using a hand treatment regularly, and that my injured nails are repaired the next morning. My favorites are Wonder-Gel Nail & Hand Exfoliating Spa Treatment, $14, and Mary Kay Satin Hands Set, $28.

The pros prove a product doesn't have to be designed for hands to do the trick. Peter Thomas Roth and June Jacobs choose one of Jacobs' luscious body products, the almost edible Lemon Sugar Scrub. Other scrubs include California North Gelskin Scrub (Jim Miller) and SkinCeuticals Body Polish (Debra Luftman). Wende Zomnir has the most unusual pick for a hand treatment—Weleda Baby Cream. Only one pro picks a product specifically designed for hands: Shauna Raisch, who chooses One Minute Manicure.

Cuticle Creams

The Buzz from the Beauty Editor

Sure, I'm beauty-obsessed, but there are a few categories even I hadn't fully explored. Cuticle creams are one of them. First of all, I don't have problematic cuticles. They are not particularly dry or stubborn or straggly. But I did have persistent hangnails, particularly on my thumbs. Researching this category took care of that problem. My husband's mother taught him this tip growing up, and it's perfect for keeping cuticles under control. After every shower, use a towel and your fingertip to keep cuticles pushed back and looking neat. (This works best on unpainted nails.) My favorite cuticle creams are Christian Dior Crème Abricot Fortifying Cream for Nails, $21, and Elizabeth Arden Eight Hour Cream Skin Protectant, $15.

What the Pros Choose

June Jacobs Cuticle Recovery Cream gets two nods (June Jacobs and Peter Thomas Roth), as does Burt's Bees Lemon Butter Cuticle Cream (Linda Deslauriers and Meredith Green). Oil lovers include Wende Zomnir (One Minute Manicure Cuticle Oil), Shauna Raisch (Solar Oil), and GIELLA (GIELLA Cuticle Clicks). Cuticle Clicks offer a customizable blend of four essential oils—kukui, avocado, grapeseed, and tea tree—to create a formula tailored to the customer's specific cuticle needs, all in a handy, mess-free pen. Top manicurists Elisa Ferri and Skyy Hadley both choose cuticle removers: Ferri picked Nailene 1-Minute Cuticle Remover, while Hadley went for Creative Nail Design AHA Cuticle Eraser.

Hand Creams

The Buzz from the Beauty Editor

I am obsessed with hand creams. I keep a tube or a pump bottle by every sink, and apply it after every hand washing. If I'm leaving the house, I replace my regular hand creams with a sunscreen, or at minimum, a hand cream with sunscreen. A dermatologist gave me the sunscreen-as-hand-cream tip, and I've never looked back. After all, the most important thing you can do to prevent aging is shield your skin from the sun, and sunscreens have plenty of emollients. My favorite hand creams are Source Ocean Hydro-Active Barrier Hand Cream, $15, H2O+ Hand and Nail Cream, $14, and No-Crack Hand Cream, $13.95.

What the Pros Choose

There is little repetition in this category. Two products are picked twice: June Jacobs Spa Collection Citrus Hand Rescue, chosen by June Jacobs and Peter Thomas Roth, and Clarins Hand and Nail Treatment Cream, the choice of Julie Hewett and Dee DeLuca-Mattos. Other picks include Santa Maria Novella Pasta di Mandorle (Meg Thompson), Ahava Advanced Hand Cream (Wende Zomnir), Fresh Milk Hand Cream (Hara Glick), Boscia Daily Hand Revival Therapy SPF15 (Meredith Green), Pure Fiji Hydrating Body Lotion in Coconut Infusion (Gabrielle Ophals), Blisslabs High Intensity Hand Cream (Skyy Hadley), Aveda Hand Relief (Shauna Raisch), and ROC Enydrial Hand Cream (Debra Luftman). Shan Albert raves about Franché CranMary Hand & Body Smoothie Lotion: "It's rich, luscious, and smells incredibly good. It contains cranberry to protect the skin and rosemary to revitalize. The ingredients are fabulous: milk extracts, shea butter, olive oil, vitamins A and E, and betafructan, which helps the skin moisturize itself. I love it because it leaves the skin feeling incredibly soft with no greasy feel."

Nail Strengtheners

The Buzz from the Beauty Editor

My nails are naturally strong and, since I don't wear them long, nail strengtheners have never been a big part of my beauty routine. I've turned to friends with chronically weak nails to compile this list. It's important to keep nails away from water, as much as possible, if weak nails are a problem. Those lame plastic kitchen gloves are your friends! Wear them when you do anything, and if you hate the way they look, get one of the newer, zippier versions, with polka dots or faux-mink trim. My top picks for strengtheners are Avon Nail Experts Strong Results Length & Strength Complex, $6, and OPI Natural Nail Strengthener, $5.95.

What the Pros Choose

OPI comes out the winner, with Meredith Green and Peter Thomas Roth putting its Natural Nail Strengthener at the top of their lists, while Shauna Raisch opts for Nail Envy. Kathryn Alice picks Tend Skin's Hard Top Nail Hardener; Dee DeLuca-Mattos loves Essie; and Elisa Ferri loves Nailene Titanium Strength. The most intriguing answer comes from Wende Zomnir: her favorite nail strengthener is "this weird, probably illegal stuff from one of my vendors that only comes off with sunscreen…don't know what's in it…don't want to know…" And the most enthusiastic answer? Skyy Hadley's pick of Trind Moisturizing Nail Balsam: "It's a product from Holland that you can get at Henri Bendel, and it's amazing. It's the perfect system. It holds moisture in the nails, which keeps them flexible and prevents them from breaking."

Nail Polish

The Buzz from the Beauty Editor

I'm not that adventurous when it comes to nail polish. I branched out a bit in the mid-nineties with Chanel Vamp, but otherwise, I tend to stick to pink-based neutrals or classic reds. They just work for me. When choosing a pale neutral polish, pay attention to the shade: many cream-colored polishes have a hint of yellow or brown that makes nails look dingy. Choose a neutral with a pink or white tone for a look that is clean and elegant.

Nails look best on the short side, squared off with rounded edges, and impeccable—I think choosing a manicurist is second in importance only to choosing a dermatologist. My favorites are Essie South of the Hi' Way, $6, OPI I'm Not Really A Waitress and Privacy Please, $6, and Chanel Pulsar, $17.

Quick-Dry Products

The Buzz from the Beauty Editor

Like many women, I never seem to wait long enough for my nail polish to dry. Regular polishes seem to take forever—that's why I love quick-dry products. They beat waiting in the salon with your hands under a dryer. Once you're in the car, direct the air conditioning vents on to your nails and they'll be dry in minutes. Also, apply another coat of your top-coat the day after your manicure, rather than waiting the standard two days. It will last much longer. My favorites are OPI DripDry, $8.75, and DeMert Nail Spray, $2.50.

What the Pros Choose

Essie is clearly a favorite among the pros. It is the polish of choice of five of our experts: June Jacobs, Hara Glick, Peter Thomas Roth, Jennifer Leung, and Dee DeLuca-Mattos. Jin Soon Choi is a fan of Essie's colors, particularly the neutrals, like Mademoiselle and Sugar Daddy. Glick's favorite is the ever-popular Ballet Slippers, while Pansy is Leung's pedicure pick. Second in line is OPI, the choice of three pros: Meredith Green, Shauna Raisch, and Meg Thompson (Cajun Shrimp). Jennifer Leung also chooses OPI Miso Happy With This Color as her top manicure shade. Chanel also gets three votes: Julie Hewett, Jennifer Leung, who picks Organdy as one of her top shades for toes, as well as Jin Soon Choi, who picks Ballerina as a favorite shade. Other picks include Hard Candy (Wende Zomnir), Trish McEvoy (Debra Luftman), and Nailene Hard & Healthy French Manicure Kit (Elisa Ferri). Jin Soon Choi also raves about NARS Nail Polish, $15: "NARS makes the best reds, and they're so popular in my salon. Jungle Red is lighter, and Chinatown is darker." The most unusual, and emphatic, choice comes from Skyy Hadley: Zoya Nail Polish, a toluene-and-formaldehyde-free formula. "If you use it, your nails will last forever," Hadley raves. "It's hard to get, but…Omigosh. It's amazing. I don't know what's in it, but it works."

What the Pros Choose

OPI wins out here, with two pros, Meredith Green and June Jacobs, choosing OPI RapiDry Top Coat as their favorite, and Shauna Raisch selecting DripDry. Debra Luftman picks Sally Hansen; Wende Zomnir likes One Minute Manicure Cuticle Oil; Dee DeLuca-Mattos chooses Out the Door; Skyy Hadley picks Seche Vite; and Gabrielle Ophals selects Qtica 1/2 Time Drying Accelerator.

Foot Creams

The Buzz from the Beauty Editor

Since I work at a computer and religiously shun exercise, my feet don't see a lot of abuse. My one foot sin: my omnipresent stilettos. All that pressure on the balls of my feet causes the skin on my soles to get dry and slightly calloused. Avoid blisters while wearing heels by applying some Sex Wax (yes, the same stuff that surfers use) to feet before slipping them into your stilettos. Miraculously, feet remain blister-free, no matter how punishing the footwear. My favorites are DDF Pedi-Cream, $24, and Peter Thomas Roth AHA Exfoliating Foot Cream, $40.

What the Pros Choose

Peter Thomas Roth singles out his AHA Exfoliating Foot Cream while also giving a nod to June Jacobs Tea Tree Foot Rescue, which is also Jacobs's pick. Other picks include Davies Gate Cardamom Foot Butter (Wende Zomnir and Gabrielle Ophals), Decleor Comfort Foot Cream (Charles Worthington), Santa Maria Novella Crema Pedestre (Meg Thompson), Aveda Foot Relief (Shauna Raisch), and Barielle Cucumber Foot Cream (Elisa Ferri). Skyy Hadley raves about Creative Nail Design Spa Pedicure Cucumber Heel Therapy: "I love this stuff. It's amazing. All you need is a dime-sized amount. You have to try it."

Appendix A

Shan Albert's Guide to Naturally Effective Anti-Aging Ingredients

ALPHA LIPOIC ACID

A powerful antioxidant that is four hundred times more potent than vitamin E and vitamin C. It is soluble in both water and lipids, which makes it able to reach and protect both the water and lipid portions of the cell. It also plays a vital role in the energy production of the cells, and helps ensure that they function at their most efficient. Alpha lipoic acid is also a potent anti-inflammatory.

AMINOGUANIDINE

An inhibitor of the advanced glycosylation pathway—a condition in which sugar irreversibly attaches to collagen, thus making the collagen fibrils brittle. The name for these sugars that attach to the proteins is advanced glycosylation endproducts, or A.G.E. Aminoguanidine is a derivative of guanidine, which is found in turnip juice, mushrooms, corn germ, rice hulls, and mussels. It short-circuits the mass crystallization (that occurs with the onset of old age) in which the skin's protein matrix suffers. Aminoguanidine helps to keep the skin soft and supple.

APPLE (PYRUS MALUS) EXTRACT

Botanical that protects against premature aging of the skin by reducing the skin-damaging effects of free radicals. Skin firming.

AVOCADO EXTRACT, SOY OIL EXTRACT

Increase collagen production and reduce inflammation.

BETA-D-GLUCOSAMINE

The most abundant of the amino sugars, which are important components of glycoproteins, glycosphingolipids, and glycosaminoglycans. Being a smaller molecule than its biochemical offspring (e.g., chitin, NaPCA, mucin), beta-glucosamine penetrates more deeply and reaches farther in its effects. Besides its role as "building block," beta-D-glucosamine is one of the many small molecular weight chemicals that makes the natural moisturizing factor (NMF). Macroscopically, beta-D-glucosamine applied topically alleviates skin dryness, facilitates exfoliation, with smoothness replacing "scales."

BLUEBERRY (VACCINIUM CORYMBOSUM L, ERICACEAE)

Contains catechin (anti-inflammatory, antioxidant, immunostimulant), alpha-carotene (pre-vitamin A), caffeic acid (anti-elastase, analgesic, antibacterial), ellagic (anti-inflammatory, antioxidant), gallic, rosmarinic, ursolic and oleanolic acids, rutin, quercitrin acid, and scopoletin.

BORAGE OIL

Very high in essential fatty acids, it is the richest known source of GLA. It has a significant effect on improving the health and appearance of skin tissue. Clinically, Borage Oil has been shown to be a very effective agent for treating skin disorders and for alleviating inflammatory symptoms associated with these disorders. It appears to positively affect the texture, suppleness, and moisture content of skin.

CASSIA BETAGLYCAN

From cassia bark. It contains D-catechin, which boosts immunity, and betaglycan, which is calming when the skin is experiencing immune reactions.

CHASTE TREE

Contains hormones that the body recognizes and can utilize. It contains 1 7-hydroxy-progesterone, delta-3-keto-steroids, and progesterone. Progesterone is metabolized in the skin like estrogen. These hormones are anti-inflammatory, they block over-keratinization, normalize pigmentation, increase the skin's natural emulsifiers to accommodate more youthful ratios of water to lipids, and, like Retin-A, they block collagenase activity.

D-BETA-FRUCTAN

From the date palm. It assists with moisture retention in the skin—just as it does with dates. The universal "drought stress" weapon in plants. Boosts immunity and builds moisture. It guides the activity of glucosamine into the cellular compartments that oversee the skin's moisture retention. In other words, it helps the skin moisturize itself.

D-BETA-GLUCOSAMINE

From Chinese foxglove, this draws moisture into collagen and elastin fibers of the skin. This sugar works to help the skin build its own stable of resident mucopolysaccharides. This right-handed chitin sugar supplies nitrogen to the skin's network of signaling molecules so that there will be accurate communication between cells. This keeps the epidermis in tighter alignment with the dermis. Together with D-beta fructan, above, it makes the effects of this arrangement more enduring. In other words, it helps strengthen the skin.

D-BOLDINE

A natural alkaloid from the Chilean boldo tree (Peumus boldus Mol). This right-handed molecule is the chirally correct form. Left-handed boldine, L-boldine, is not present in the boldo tree. It is only present in synthetic boldine. L-boldine is not good for the body but D-boldine is very good for it. D-boldine protects the cells, is anti-inflammatory, is a powerful antioxidant and prevents peroxidation, and is very calming.

D-QUERCETIN/URSOLIC ACID

Derived from evening primrose, it is the way quercetin and ursolic exist together—it is the chirally correct form (left-handed) and the most effective. This flavonoid provides a yellow or gold color to a formulation while also being a powerful antioxidant, anti-peroxidant, and anti-inflammatory. Research of D-quercetin has shown that it has the following abilities and properties*:

- Analgesic
- Anti-allergenic
- Antibacterial
- Anti-herpes
- Anti-HIV
- Anti-psoriasis
- Cancer preventative
- Protects capillaries

* D-Qu (D-quercetin) is a bioflavonoid and is used both topically and internally. It is the most abundant of the flavonoid molecules. Quercetin has also shown potent anti-cancer activity. Quercetin has "been shown to inhibit the growth of cells derived from human and animal cancers, such as leukemia and Ehrlich ascites tumors, the estrogen receptor-positive breast carcinoma (MCF-7), squamous cell carcinoma of head and neck origin, gastric cancer and colon cancer, as well as human leukemia HL-60 cells in culture [Vang et al reported resveratrol to be active in normalizing HL-60 cells in culture back into normal cells]. . . . Quercetin has antiproliferative activity against breast and stomach cancer cell lines and human ovarian cancer primary cultures and can potentiate the action of [the anti-cancer drug] cisplatin ex vivo. . . . Hoffman et al in 1988 related both quercetin's direct anti-cancer activity, as well as its synergistic effect with several standard anti-cancer drugs to its ability to inhibit the enzyme protein kinase C." They also noted that Quercetin "…is a licensed [anti-cancer] drug in many countries, and is non-toxic at the required dose range." Also, go to http://jac.oxfordjournals.org/cgi/content/full/52/2/194 and you'll be able to read more about studies involving quercetin and anti-viral activities (including herpes and HIV). Be sure to scroll down.

ENZYMES (FRUIT, PLANT, AND VEGETABLE)

Pineapple fruit and stem and Spanish moss enzymes are exfoliating as well as being anti-inflammatory. When properly processed, pumpkin enzymes, rich in vitamin A and other vitamins and minerals, produce a good amount of exfoliation. Papaya is also an excellent exfoliant, and so is cranberry. The D-complex of cranberry is rich in vaccinin, a biomolecular "vaccine" against viruses, bacteria, and fungus. Cranberry also contains D-gamma-tocopherol, which has the ability to keep skin cells "fertile" for self-renewal.

HYALURONIC ACID

Hyaluronic acid is a natural polysaccharide formed by the sugars N-acetyl-D-glucosamine and glucuronic acid in very long chains, a structure which is similar in bacteria, animals, and humans. In animals, the main biologic function of hyaluronic acid is in connective tissue, stabilizing the intercellular structures and forming the matrix in which collagen and elastin fibers are embedded. In young skin, it is found at the periphery and interfaces of collagen and elastin fibers, helping to hold them together in the proper configuration. These connections with hyaluronic acid seem to be absent in aged skin, one possible factor in the disorganization of collagen and elastin fibers. Hyaluronic acid decreases with photoaging, a decrease that may be partly responsible for wrinkles and loss of plumpness because together with this loss we lose water retention. Hyaluronic acid's water-binding ability makes it a great humectant and moisturizing ingredient for skin care products; it has the ability to pull moisture from the atmosphere and trap it on the surface of the skin, and it has been shown to penetrate the stratum corneum and enter the epidermis. It will also replenish the sugars required to make new hyaluronic acid in the dermis. Recently, topical products have been launched that intend to capitalize on the popularity of the new dermal fillers that contain cross linked hyaluronic acid. This is a bit like the "better than Botox" campaigns that promise Botox effects without the pain or the cost, but hyaluronic acid applied topically will not have a filler effect like that provided by injections of cross-linked hyaluronic acid. The skin layer is not cells but proteins (like collagen and elastin) in a matrix that has glycoproteins (fibronectin, tenascin), glycosaminoglycans (hyaluronic acid, dermatan sulfate, and others), and water. Hyaluronic acid is thought to be the main water-regulating molecule in this matrix.

L-ALPHA BISABOLOL

From chamomile, this is the left-handed, chirally correct form of bisabolol. It is far better than azulene as an anti-inflammatory, wound healer, and anti-burn ingredient.

L-ASCORBIC ACID

This is the chirally correct vitamin C, and is an antioxidant and a cofactor for an enzyme crucial in the synthesis of collagen. Vitamin C scavenges and destroys reactive oxidizing agents and other free radicals. Because of this ability, it provides important protection against damage induced by UV radiation (and the DNA mutations and cancer that may result from it). Vitamin C also improves skin elasticity, decreases wrinkles by stimulating collagen synthesis, reduces erythema, promotes wound healing, and suppresses cutaneous pigmentation. Because body control mechanisms limit the amount of ingested vitamin C available to skin, topical antioxidant therapy becomes an attractive way to target vitamin C directly into skin. Products containing vitamin C should be protected from light and containers should be closed carefully after each use.

L-LACTIC ACID

A left-handed, chirally correct AHA which is better accepted by the skin than any other. It exfoliates with less stress to the skin. Protein-softening and stimulates cell turnover. Its effects on the skin are very similar to glycolic acid polymer. It promotes healthier growth of new skin and more accurate differentiation of cells. It also keeps glucose from attaching to protein sites, thus helping to keep the skin soft and supple.

L-RETINOL AGP

A left-handed, chirally correct vitamin-A complex. The benefits of retinol are enhanced by complexing it with AGP (arabinogalactan protein conjugates). AGP is derived from wine and is an important part of what makes wine healthy. Other important components of AGP are glucuronic acid and praline. Both are important to the health of the body and especially the skin.

LIQUID CRYSTALS

Derived from plant cells, they strengthen the cell wall and help plug up any leaks, thereby helping the cell to maintain the proper fluid levels. This in turn keeps the cell firm.

MANGO

Mangifera indica use dates back to at least four thousand years ago in India and twenty-five hundred years ago in Southeast Asia. The Portuguese introduced mango to Brazil during the early 1700s, and its cultivation spread to the West Indies. Mango is one of those plants that merit the use of whole fruit extract rather than a fraction enriched in a particular chemical. This is because mango contains so many beneficial chemicals:

- Fruit acids (citric, ascorbic, malic) for mild exfoliation
- Gallic acid (analgesic, antiviral, antibacterial, antimutagenic, anti-inflammatory)
- Kaempferol (phytoestrogen, antiallergic, anticancer, antibacterial, anti-inflammatory, antiviral)
- Lauric acid (antibacterial, antiviral)
- Myristic acid (cancer preventive)
- Quercetin (antiviral, antibacterial, antioxidant, antipsoriatic)
- Ascorbic acid (vitamin C, essential to skin metabolism, stimulates collagen synthesis)
- Carotenoids
- Catalase
- Peroxidase
- Essential fatty acids (linoleic acid, linolenic acid)
- Vitamins (C, B6, niacin, pantothenic acid)
- Amino acids
- Minerals (silica, sulfur, copper, zinc, and boron, which are required for the activity of important skin enzymes)

POLYPEPTIDES

These are considered to be the newest find in anti-aging ingredients. Amino acids are the subunits that make up a protein. Although there are many amino acids, only twenty (all of them with L-chirality) are common in proteins. Amino acids can join each other in a peptide bond. Two amino acids joined in a peptide bond constitute a dipeptide, three a tripeptide, a few an oligopeptide, and many a polypeptide. A protein can be made up of just one or several polypeptides. In the cosmetic industry, we use many different proteins, like collagen or elastin, and proteins with enzymatic activity, like papain or superoxide dismutase. Recently, the industry started using synthetic peptides, made to mimic peptides found to have beneficial activity on the skin. For example, there is a tripeptide, glycyl-histidyl-lysine, that is good at carrying copper and has been shown to help with wound healing (no effect has been demonstrated on skin aging).

Palmitoyl pentapeptide (trademarked as Matrixyl) is a fatty-acid derivative of a synthetic pentapeptide, KTTKS (the names of amino acids can be abbreviated as one or three letters). There are no independent studies on the effectiveness of this peptide on skin aging—only those done by the researchers who developed it. Matrixyl was developed by Parisian researchers and is made up of a patented blend of water-soluble molecules, five amino acids (called peptides), and proteoglycans (MatrixylR 1999). This combination lends much-needed support to the collagen/elastin matrix that helps keep skin firm, resilient, and smooth-feeling. Together, this blend forms a gel that encourages mature skin cells to produce fresh new skin tissue that can push out and replace dead cells.

Another peptide example is EEMQRR (trademarked as Argireline). Again, the evidence is not very firm. On the other hand, it is likely that all of these peptides benefit the skin in one way or another. The problem is that synthetic peptides are very expensive and manufacturers may use very little in their formulas. Marine oligopeptides are natural polypeptides obtained from a natural source. Because of their relatively low price, they can be added in concentrations that will ensure not just good copper transport, but also provide the skin the amino acids it needs to make its own collagen and even help the skin retain moisture. The copper source is copper gluconate, which is added in very small amounts, as copper is essential but can be toxic in high concentrations.

RESVERATROL

Resveratrol (3,5,4'-trans-trihydroxystilbene) is found in some higher plants like Vitis vinifera (mostly in the red-grape varieties), pine nuts, and in very high concentrations in the root of *Polygonum cuspidatum*. In the plant its function seems to be that of a messenger that activates a series of defensive mechanisms. Stress, be it a viral infection (plants can also be infected by viruses, bacteria, and fungi) or UV irradiation, induces its synthesis. And what can resveratrol do for humans? Epidemiological studies showed that French people, despite being so fond of cooking with butter and cream, have a relatively low incidence of cardiac disease. Why? The secret of the so-called French paradox—the resveratrol present in the glass of red wine the French like to have with their meals. Resveratrol can also help in the treatment of skin problems caused by stress. Resveratrol properties are many: antioxidant, radical scavenger, anti-inflammatory, vasodilator, stimulates cellular proliferation and collagen synthesis, inhibits proteases, and blocks the deleterious effects from UVB radiation.

RETINOL (VITAMIN A)

This helps bring any type of skin back to a normal pH level and balance. It has the ability to penetrate the skin and increase its elasticity. It can also thicken the epidermis and dermis and increase cell turnover.

ROSEMARY

Rosemary contains L-carnesol, which is an anti-inflammatory and antioxidant, and L-hesperidin, also an anti-inflammatory and antioxidant as well as a counter-irritant.

SALICYLIC ACID

From pumpkin seeds, it is great for sloughing off dead skin cells and is very effective in reversing the visible signs of aging when combined with glycolic or lactic acid. It is also a potent anti-inflammatory and a natural spin trap (see below).

SHEA BUTTER

From the fruit of the karite tree, its L-phytosterols and D-alpha tocopherol prevent lipid peroxidation in epidermis. It's soothing and an anti-inflammatory. Ideally, shea butter is combined with antioxidants and growth factors, or exfoliants, if it is to be part of an anti-aging formula.

SPIN TRAP

A form of nitrogen, it is often called the intelligent antioxidant because it only targets the out-of-control free radicals that are doing damage. It stops the out-of-control spin and leads the oxygen free radicals back into the respiratory cycle where they belong.

THIOREDOXIN

This can be derived from yeast, and is part of the antioxidant system that protects most living beings from damage inflicted by our highly oxidant environment, an atmosphere with 21 percent oxygen and UV rays that start cascades producing a multitude of free radicals. We depend on oxygen for respiration, but are also damaged by oxygen and the by-products of respiration itself. Damage by free radicals formed in response to UV light is now believed to be a major cause of skin aging, with the term photo-aging being used to describe the effect of sunlight on the skin. Topical application of Thioredoxin should be able to prevent some of this damage.

Appendix B

Shan Albert's Guide to Naturally Effective Anti-Acne Ingredients

AZELAIC ACID

Azelaic acid occurs naturally in potato tubers, grains, etc. It breaks down and removes the dead cells on the skin surface. It also kills bacteria on the skin. Azelaic acid has been shown to be effective in the treatment of hyperpigmentation (including melasma). It is at least as effective as hydroquinone but is less irritating and much better tolerated. This is beneficial in reducing the discolorations left by acne blemishes. Azelaic acid is effective in the treatment of comedonal and inflammatory acne, where it has been shown to be as effective as topical tretinoin, benzoyl peroxide, erythromycin, and oral tetracycline. Azelaic acid will also loosen the keratinocytes, decreasing the likelihood of comedone (blackhead) formation. In addition, Azelaic acid has been shown to be effective in the treatment of rosacea and has anti-tumorigenic power.

B VITAMINS

Anti-stress vitamins. Soothing. Acneic skin is usually very irritated and needs to be calmed and soothed.

BENZOYL PEROXIDE

Benzoyl peroxide is effective, but it is a strong oxidizer and will form oxygen radicals. It is very effective in killing Propionibacterium acnes, and it has some effect on microcomedo formation. But it will often cause erythema (redness of the skin produced by congestion of the capillaries), scaling, and sometimes contact sensitivity. Possible alternative: retinoids, which will do a much better job of preventing the formation of microcomedos. A large number of ingredients will kill P. acnes, among them Totarol and tea tree oil.

BISMUTH OXYCHOLIDE

A mineral derived from the earth's crust, this soothes and heals. It is also anti-inflammatory and oil absorbing.

CHOLIC ACID

Plant-based acid that reduces sebum production and helps to thin sebum.

CRANBERRY (VACCINIUM MACROCARPON: ERICACEAE)

Contains Alpha-terpineol (anti-acne, antiseptic, healing), anthocyanosides, benzoic acid (antiseptic), lutein (cancer preventive), quercetin, and vitamin B-6. Cranberry (*Vaccinium macrocarpon*) contains an amazing array of beneficial chemicals. The procyanidins, leucocyanin and leucodelphinin, and flavonol glucosides, including myricetin-3-pyranoside, inhibit bacterial adhesion; their net effect is to inhibit bacterial growth. In addition, several quercetin and myricetin glycosides have potent antioxidant and free-radical scavenging activity.

EUCALYPTUS

Excellent antiseptic.

L-ALPHA BISABOLOL

From chamomile. It is the strongest part of chamomile and far better than azulene as an anti-inflammatory and wound healer.

L-LACTIC ACID

AHA exfoliant. Loosens dead skin cells and softens debris in pores. Acneic skin tends to have a buildup of dead skin cells—often "glued down" by an overabundance of sebum (oil). Removing those dead skin cells and softening the debris in the pores is a good way to assist the skin in combating acne.

NIACINAMIDE

Topical application of Niacinamide will decrease pruritus and inflammation, help acne-affected skin, decrease oiliness, alleviate atopic dermatitis, decrease UV-induced skin cancers, and help decrease facial pigmentation.

PREGNENOLONE

Hormone precursor from plants that blocks testosterone's effect on the sebaceous gland (anti-sebum means less oil production).

PROPOLIS

From bees. The most natural antibiotic, Propolis is now considered a natural cure by the World Health Organization.

RASPBERRY

Many beneficial chemicals are derived from raspberry (Rubus idaeus) extract, including caffeic acid (analgesic, antibacterial, antimutagenic), ellagic acid (antibacterial, anti-inflammatory), ferulic acid (antibacterial, anti-inflammatory), and lutein (antioxidant).

RETINOL

Vitamin A. Infection fighter. Increases cell turnover and encourages the growth of healthy cells deep within the dermis. Controls oil.

SALICYLIC ACID

Beta Hydroxy Acid (BHA) which can be derived from pumpkin seeds. Excellent exfoliator; helps control oil and dead skin cell buildup.

TEA TREE OIL

Anti-inflammatory, antibacterial, anti-fungal, anti-tumor, anti-viral, wound healer.

TOTAROL

A naturally occurring plant extract with potent antibacterial and antioxidant properties. Thoroughly purified after extraction from the Totara (Podocarpus sp.), a giant tree in New Zealand, Totarol is a potent antioxidant with antimicrobial activity. Propionibacterium acne, the bacterium involved in acne, is particularly sensitive to this extract. Totarol is effective in the treatment of acne and rosacea.

WITCH HAZEL (HAMAMELIS VIRGINIANA)

Witch Hazel has a long history of traditional medicinal uses. It is a pharmacy in a single extract, full of chemicals that carry the following properties: antihistaminic, antiallergic, immunomodulator, analgesic, antioxidant, anti-inflammatory, antiviral, astringent, antielastase, antibacterial, antiseptic, capilliariprotective, cancer preventive, antileukotriene, and more. The chemicals responsible for these properties are ellagitannin, gallic acid, quercetin, isoquercitrin, kaempferol, L-epigallocatechin, leucocyanidin, leucodelphinidin, myricetin, quercitrin, saponins, and others.

ZEOLITE

A natural mineral that traps biological and environmental waste.

Appendix C

Glossary

A

Accutane: A trademark name for isotretinoin, a vitamin-A derivative, which is used to treat severe acne. It inhibits sebaceous gland secretion.

Acetylcholine: The first neurotransmitter ever identified.

Alpha hydroxy acid: Various fruit acids that are capable of trapping moisture in the skin and initiating the formation of collagen.

Amphoteric AHA: A form of alpha hydroxy acid which allows for slower penetration, decreasing irritation and making it more suited for sensitive skin.

Androgens: General term for any male hormone, like testosterone.

Antibiotic: A drug that kills bacteria and other germs.

Antioxidant: A chemical that inhibits oxidation.

Arginine: An amino acid found in proteins that is essential for nutrition.

Avobenzone (Parsol 1789): A sunscreen ingredient that blocks the entire spectrum of UVA radiation. Parsol 1789 is the trade name for avobenzone.

Azelaic Acid (Azelex): A naturally occurring dicarboxylic acid found in whole-grain cereals that is commonly used to treat acne and as a skin lightener.

B

Benzophenone: Benzoic acid. Commonly used in sunscreens.

Benzoyl peroxide: An antibacterial medication used to treat acne.

Beta hydroxy acid: Includes salicylic acid. Penetrates deeply to exfoliate skin.

Blepharoplasty: Eyelid surgery to remove excess fat, skin, and muscle from lower and upper eyelids, improving the appearance of the eye area.

Broad spectrum: A sunscreen that protects skin from both UVA and UVB rays.

C

Chirally correct: A product or ingredient which has the most beneficial effects with the fewest negative effects.

Coenzyme Q10: An antioxidant which inhibits the aging process on a cellular level.

D

Diuretic spironolactone: A potassium-sparing diuretic.

E

Emblica: Commonly known as the gooseberry, it is the richest known source of vitamin C.

Endermologie: A cellulite treatment using a computerized machine to massage tissues under suction.

Epidermal Growth Factor (EGF): A small protein that can help with normal cell growth and wound healing.

Essential oil: A concentrated, hydrophobic liquid containing volatile aromatic compounds extracted from plants.

F

Fraxel laser: A laser therapy which reduces fine lines and wrinkles and improves skin texture and pigmentation.

G

Genestein: One of the isoflavone class of flavonoids.

Glycolic acid peel: A skin treatment using glycolic acid to superficial wrinkles, uneven skintone, enlarged pores, acne scars, and age spots.

H

Home peel: A chemical peel that is designed for home use. It is generally milder than a professional peel.

Hydroquinone: A topical treatment designed to lighten darkened skin (from melasma, age spots, freckles, and cholasma) while decreasing the formation of melanin.

Hyperpigmentation: Darkening of the skin, commonly produced by ultraviolet radiation, which provokes melanocytes in the skin.

Hypopigmentation: A condition caused by a deficiency in melanin formation or a loss of pre-existing melanin or melanocytes.

I

Intense Pulsed Light (Photofacial): A therapy that emits high intensity pulses of light generally used for skin rejuvenation and acne treatment.

J

Jessner peel (or Jessner's peel): A peel consisting of lactic acid and salicylic acid used to lighten hyperpigmentation and to treat sun damage.

K

Kojic acid: A skin-lightening agent used to treat hyperpigmentation.

L

L-lactic acid: An AHA derived from milk, which helps skin be more flexible, smoother, and more even-toned.

Lentigines: Also known as sun spots, age spots, and liver spots. Harmless flat brown discolorations on the skin of the face, neck, and hands.

M

Melasma: Dark brown symmetrical patches of pigment on the face. Occurs in almost half of all pregnant women.

Microdermabrasion: An exfoliating treatment in which the skin is "sandblasted" with ultra-fine crystals of aluminum-oxide or other ingredients to remove the top layer of skin.

Milia (milium): Benign, keratin-filled cysts that look like tiny hard white bumps. Most commonly found around the nose or eyes.

N

Nd: Yag laser: One of the most common types of lasers used to treat a variety of skin conditions.

Neti pot: Jala neti is a yoga technique, meaning "water cleansing." Salted water is used to rinse out the nasal cavity. Also known as nasal irrigation.

O

Octyl methoxycinnamate (Parsol MCX): A common sunscreen which absorbs UVB rays

P

Parabens: A group of preservatives used in cosmetics to prevent bacterial and fungal growth in products.

Peptides: Short chains of amino acids that combine to form proteins.

Prevage: A topical antioxidant. Trade name for idebenone.

Pulsed dye laser: A laser therapy which can improve acne scarring and fine wrinkles by increasing collagen production.

R

Renova: A retinoid used to treat photo damage and hyperpigmentation.

Retin-A: A retinoid that is used as a topical prescription acne treatment.

Retinoid (Retin-A, Renova, Avage, and Differin): A vitamin-A derivative which works to increase cell turnover and exfoliation by stimulating cell production underneath the skin

Retinol: An over-the-counter vitamin-A derivative.

Rosacea: A skin condition characterized by inflamed, red, oily, acne-prone areas.

S

Salicylic acid: A drug that removes the outer layer of skin. Used to treat various skin conditions.

Stratum corneum: Outermost layer of dead cells in the epidermis.

Systemic Antibiotics: Target the bacteria P. acnes that are thought to be responsible for local infection in acne. Common antibiotics are tetracycline, erythromycin, doxycycline, and minocycline.

T

TCA peel: A trichloro acetic acid peel is a medium peel which improves superficial discoloration and eliminates fine wrinkles.

Telangiectasia: Dilated superficial blood vessels which may occur in rosacea.

Tetracycline: A systemic antibiotic used in the treatment of acne.

Titanium dioxide: A physical sunscreen that acts as a sun block. It will not break down in the heat.

Tretinoin/Retinoic Acid: A vitamin-A derivative used to treat acne.

Triactive: A laser treatment which can temporarily reduce the appearance of cellulite.

U

UVA (Ultraviolet A): Long wave solar rays responsible for wrinkles and photoaging, resulting in a leathery appearance.

UVB (Ultraviolet B): Short wave solar rays responsible for sunburn and skin cancer.

V

Vitamin K: A vitamin that acts to protect our body from bleeding problems. In skin care, it is used to treat bruises and spider veins.

Z

Zinc oxide: A physical sunblock that soothes and protects against UVA/UVB rays.

Appendix D

Shopping Guide

A

A&D Baby Ointment: drug and discount stores nationwide
Acqua Di Parma: www.acquadiparma.it
Ahava: www.AhavaUS.com
Air Stocking: www.bellneusa.com
Almay: www.almay.com; drug and discount stores nationwide
Alpha Hydrox: www.alphahydrox.com
Amanda Lacey: www.amandalacey.com
Anastasia: www.anastasia.net
Anna Sui: www.annasuibeauty.com
Anthony Morrocco: www.morroccomethod.com
Aquaphor: www.eucerin.com; drug and discount stores nationwide
Archipelago Botanicals: www.archipelago-usa.com
Arrojo Studio: www.arrojostudio.com
ARTec: salons nationwide
As U Wish Nail Spa: www.asuwishnailspa.com
Avance: www.avanceskincare.com

Aveda: www.aveda.com
Aveeno: www.aveeno.com; drug and discount stores nationwide
Avon: www.avon.com
Awake: www.awakecosmetics.com

B

B. Kamins: www.bkamins.com
Baby Magic: www.babymagic.com
Bare Escentuals: www.bareescentuals.com
Barielle: www.barielle.com
Bath & Body Works: www.bathandbodyworks.com
Bath by Bettijo: www.bathbybettijo.com
Beauticontrol: www.beauticontrol.com
Becca: www.beccacosmetics.com
Benefit: www.benefitcosmetics.com
Beyond Spa: www.humc.com/beyond
Bior: www.juliehewett.net
Biotherm: www.biotherm-usa.com
Biotone: www.biotone.com

Black Opal: www.blackopalbeauty.com

Blinc: www.blincinc.com

Bliss: www.blissworld.com

Blistex: www.blistex.com; drug and discount stores nationwide

Bloom: www.bloomcosmetics.com

Blue Cross: beauty supply stores

Bobbe Joy: www.bobbejoycosmetics.com

Bobbi Brown: www.bobbibrowncosmetics.com

Bonne Bell: www.bonnebell.com; drug and discount stores nationwide

Boscia: www.boscia.net

BridalGal: www.bridalgal.com

Bumble and bumble: www.bumbleandbumble.com

Burt's Bees: www.burtsbees.com

Butterfly Studio Salon: www.butterflystudiosalon.com

C

California Baby: www.californiababy.com

California North: www.californianorth.com

California Tan: www.californiatan.com

CARGO: www.cargocosmetics.com

Caron: 212.319.4888

Caswell-Massey: www.caswellmassey.com

Catherine Atzen: www.atzen.com

Caudalie: www.caudalie.com

Cellulite Rx: www.celluliterx.biz

Cetaphil: www.cetaphil.com

Chanel: www.chanel.com

Chantecaille: www.chantecaille.com

Chapstick: www.chapstick.com; drug and discount stores nationwide

Charles Worthington: www.charlesworthington.com

Chop Chop Salon: www.chopchopsalon.com

Cinema Secrets: www.cinemasecrets.com

Clairol: beauty supply stores nationwide

Clarins: www.clarins.com

Classified Cosmetics: www.classifiedcosmetics.com

Cle de Peau Beauté: www.sca.shiseido.com/cledepeau

Clearasil: www.clearasil.com; drug and discount stores nationwide

Clinique: www.clinique.com

Colorescience: www.colorescience.com

Colormark: www.colormarkpro.com

Cosmedix: www.cosmedix.com

Cover Girl: www.covergirl.com

Creative Nail Design: www.creativenaildesign.com

Crede: www.joybeauty.com

Curlfriends: www.curlfriends.com

D

Daniello: www.danielloskincare.com

Davies Gate: www.daviesgate.com

DDF: www.ddf.com

Debra B. Luftman, MD: www.drluftman.com

Debra Macki: www.debramacki.com

Decleor: www.decleor.com

Delux Beauty: www.deluxbeauty.com

Demert: beauty supply stores nationwide

Dermalogica: www.dermalogica.com

Dermanew: www.dermanew.com

Dior: www.dior.com

Dirty Girl: www.blueq.com

Dominique Salon: www.dominiquesalon.com

Dr. Brandt Skincare: www.drbrandtskincare.com

Dr. Hauschka: www.drhauschka.com

Dr. Jessica Wu Cosmeceuticals: www.drjessicawu.com

Dr. Mary Lupo Skin Care Systems: www.drmarylupo.com

DuWop: www.duwop.com

E

Earth Therapeutics: www.earththerapeutics.com
Ecru New York: www.ecrunewyork.com
EI Solutions: www.sephora.com
Elizabeth Arden: www.elizabetharden.com
Enessa: www.enessa.com
Epione: www.Epione.com
Essie: www.essie.com
Eve Lom: www.evelom.com

F

Face Stockholm: www.facestockholm.com
Fake Bake: www.fakebake.com
Flowery: www.flowery.com
Franché: www.franche.com
Frédéric Fekkai: www.fredericfekkai.com
Fresh: www.fresh.com
FX Special Effects: drug and discount stores nation-
    wide

G

G Spa: www.gspa.biz
GIELLA: www.giella.com
Giorgio Armani: www.giorgioarmanibeauty.com
Girlactik: www.girlactik.com
Graham Webb: www.grahamwebb.com

H

H2O Plus: www.h2oplus.com
Hair Garden: www.hairgarden.com
Hair Light: www.folica.com
Hamadi: www.hamadibeauty.com
Hard Candy: www.hardcandy.com
Haven: www.havensoho.com
Henri Bendel: www.bathandbodyworks.com

I

Il Makiage: www.il-makiage.com
In Fiore: www.beautyhabit.com
ISH: www.ishrescue.com
Issimo: www.issimointernational.com

J

J. Beverly Hills: www.jbeverlyhills.com
Jan Marini Skin Research: www.janmarini.com
Jane Iredale: www.janeiredale.com
Janet Sartin: www.sartin.com
Jessica Cosmetics: www.jessicacosmetics.com
Jo Malone: www.jomalone.com
Joe Blasco: www.joeblasco.com
John Frieda: www.johnfrieda.com; drug and discount
    stores nationwide
John Ivey, DMD: www.johniveydmd.com
Jonathan Product: www.jonathanproduct.com
Julie Hewett: www.juliehewett.net
Julien Farel Salon: www.julienfarel.com
June Jacobs: www.junejacobs.com

K

Kerastase: www.kerastase-usa.com
Keri: www.kerilotion.com; drug and discount
    stores nationwide
Kett Cosmetics: www.kettcosmetics.com
Kiehl's: www.kiehls.com
Kinara Spa: www.kinaraspa.com
Kinerase: www.kinerase.com
Komenuka-Bijin: www.komenuka-Bijin.com

L

L'Occitane: www.loccitane.com
L'Oreal: www.loreal.com; drug and discount stores
    nationwide

La Bella Donna: www.labelladonna.com
La Mer: www.cremedelamer.com
La Prairie: www.laprairie.com
La Roche Posay: www.laroche-posay.us
Lamas Beauty: www.lamasbeauty.com
Lancôme: www.Lancôme.com
Lansinoh: www.lansinoh.com
Laura Mercier: www.lauramercier.com
Lava: www.wd40.com
Lavande Nail Spa: www.lavandenailspa.com
Lavera: www.lavera-usa.com
Le Salon Chinois: www.lesalonchinois.com
Leaf & Rusher: www.leafandrusher.com
Lipsense: www.senegence.com
Lola: www.lolacosmetics.com
LORAC: www.loraccosmetics.com
Love Nectar Potions Honey Rose Kissing Balm:
      www.celebrationsoflove.com
Lucky Chick: www.luckychick.com
LUSH: www.lush.com

M

MAC: www.maccosmetics.com
Madge: www.madgecosmetics.com
Magic Tan: www.magictanexperience.com
Make Up For Ever: www.makeupforever.com
Makeover Specialist: www.makeoverspecialist.com
Makeup Alley: www.makeupalley.com
Mario Russo: www.mariorusso.com
Martina Gebhardt Naturkosmetik:
      www.martina-gebhardt-naturkosmetik.de/;
      health food stores nationwide
Mary Kay: www.MaryKay.com
Matrix: www.matrix.com
Max Factor: www.maxfactor.com; drug and discount
      stores nationwide
Maybelline: www.maybelline.com
MD Formulations: www.mdformulations.com

MD Forté: www.mdforte.com
MD Skincare: www.mdskincare.com
Miano Viél Salon & Spa: www.mianoviel.com
Mode de Vie: www.modedevie.com
Modern Organic Products: www.mopproducts.com
Murad: www.murad.com
Murray's Pomade: www.murrayspomade.com
Mystic Tan: www.mystictan.com

N

Nailene: www.nailene.com
Nailtiques: www.nailtiques.com
Naked Kiss: www.tabercoinc.com
Napoleon Perdis: www.napoleonperdis.com
NARS: www.narscosmetics.com
Nelson Chan: www.nelsonchanonline.com
Neostrata: www.neostrata.com
Neutrogena: www.neutrogena.com; drug and dis-
      count stores nationwide
New York Color: www.newyorkcolor.com
Nioxin: www.nioxin.com
No-Crack: www.nocrack.com

O

Olay: www.olay.com
One Minute Manicure:
      www.oneminutemanicure.com
OPI: www.opi.com
Oribe: www.oribesalon.com
Origins: www.origins.com
Orly: www.orlybeauty.com
Osmotics: www.osmotics.com
Ouidad: www.ouidad.com
Out the Door: www.inmcanada.com; drug and
      beauty supply stores

P

Palmer's: www.etbrowne.com

Pantene: www.pantene.com; drug and discount stores nationwide

Paul & Joe: www.paul-joe-beaute.com; Sephora

Paul Brown: www.paulbrownhawaii.com

Paul Mitchell: www.paulmitchell.com

Paula Dorf: www.pauladorf.com

Peter Thomas Roth: www.peterthomasroth.com

Pevonia: www. pevonia.com

Pharmaskincare: www.pharmaskincare.com

Philosophy: www.philosophy.com

Physicians Formula: www.physiciansformula.com; drug and discount stores nationwide

Phytotherathrie: www.phytotherathrie.com

Pierre Michel: www.pierremichelbeauty.com

Pop Beauty: www.popbeauty.co.uk/; Sephora

Pout: Sephora

Prada Beauty: Neiman Marcus

Prescriptives: www.prescriptives.com

Pretty Pretty: www.pretty2.com

Prevage: www.prevage.com

Prive: www.priveproducts.com

Proactiv Solution: proactiv.com

Pur Minerals: www.purminerals.com

Pure Fiji: www.purefiji.com

Pureology: www.pureology.com

Q

Qtica: www.qtica.com; www.artofbeauty.com

R

Redken: www.redken.com

Rene Furterer: www.renefurterer.com

Revercel: www.revercel.com

Revlon: www.revlon.com; drug and discount stores nationwide

Ric Pipino: www.pipino.com

Robert Kree: www.robertkree.com

ROC: www.rocskincare.com; drug and discount stores nationwide

S

Sally Hansen: www.sallyhansen.com; drug and discount stores nationwide

Santa Maria Novella: www.lafcony.com

Schwarzkopf: www.schwarzkopf.com

Sea Breeze: drug and discount stores nationwide

Sebastian Trucco: www.sebastian-intl.com

Seche Vite: www.seche.com

Seki Edge: www.sekiedge.com

Sephora: www.sephora.com

Sexy Hair Concepts: www.sexyhairconcepts.com

Shinbi: www.diamondbeauty.com

Shiseido: www.shiseido.co.jp/com

Shu Uemura: www.shuuemura-usa.com

Sircuit Cosmeceuticals: www.sircuitskin.com

Sisley: Neiman Marcus

Själ: www.isjal.com

Skin Effects by Dr. Jeffrey Dover: www.cvs.com; CVS stores nationwide

Skinceuticals: www.skinceuticals.com

Skingenious: www.skingenious.com

Smashbox: www.smashbox.com

Smith's Rosebud Salve: www.sephora.com

Sonya Dakar: www.SonyaDakar.com

Source Ocean: www.sourceocean.com

St. Tropez: www.sttropeztan.com

Stephane Marais: www.stephanemarais.com

Stephen Sollitto: www.sollitto.net

Stila: www.Stilacosmetics.com

Sudzz FX: www.sudzzfx.com

Sue Devitt: www.suedevittstudio.com

Sun: www.sunlaboratories.com

Sundari: www.sundari.com

Swabplus: www.swabplus.com

T

T. LeClerc: www.t-leclerc.com

Tammy Taylor Natural Nail Shaper: www.tammytay-lornails.com

Tan Towels: www.tantowel.com

Tarte: www.TarteCosmetics.com

Tend Skin: www.tendskin.com

Terax: www.teraxhaircare.com

The Balm: www.thebalm.com

The Organic Bath Co.: www.organicbathco.com

The Organic Sudz Company: www.kissmyface.com

The Thymes Ltd.: www.thymes.com

The Vital Image: www.thevitalimage.com

TIGI: www.tigihaircare.com

Tina Earnshaw: www.tinaearnshaw.com

Tresemmé: www.tresemme.com

Trind: www.trindusa.com

Trish McEvoy: www.trishmcevoy.com

Tweezerman: tweezerman.com

Twiggs Salonspa: www.twiggssalonspa.com

U

Urban Decay: www.urbandecay.com

V

Valmont: www.valmont.ch/products

Victoria's Secret: www.victoriassecret.com; Victoria's Secret stores nationwide

Vincent Longo: www.vincentlongo.com

W

Weleda: usa.weleda.com

Wella: www.wellausa.com

Wellbox: www.wellbox.com

Wet 'n Wild: www.wetnwild.com

Wonder-Gel: www.the-spa-authority.com

Y

YG Laboratories: www.yglabs.com

Yon-Ka: www.yonka.com

Yuko Systems: www.yukobeauty.com

Yves Saint Laurent: www.ysl.com; Neiman Marcus, Bergdorf Goodman

Z

Z. Bigatti: www.zbigatti.com

Zoya: www.zoya.com; www.artofbeauty.com

Index

Blisters. *See* Feet

Blondes, 151–152

    brassiness, 152

    green tint, 153–154

Blow-dryers, 133–134

Blueberry (Vaccinium corymbosum L // Ericaceae), usage, 190

Blushes, 48–50

    mistakes, 48–49

    products, professional selection, 52

    selection, 50

        advice, 48

Blushing

    basics, 48

    beauty, 49

    process, 48

Boatner, Kari, xii, 35, 53, 68, 83

Body

    brushing, 96–97

    care, 95–98

    creams, products (professional selection), 106

    lotions, products (professional selection), 105

    shimmer/glitter, 96

    treatments, 102

    washes, products (professional selection), 103

Bojkovic, Spresa, xii, 146

Borage oil, usage, 190

BP. *See* Benzoyl peroxide

Breakouts, BP (usage), 19

Brighteners. *See* Skin

Broad spectrum, definition, 202

Bronzers

    advice, 42

    blushers, combination, 49

    definition, 43

    problems, 41–42

    products, 51–52

        professional selection, 52

    purchase, 41

Brown spots

    cessation, 112

    reduction, 24

Browning, Danielle, xii, 2

Bruising, treatment, 97

Brunette hair, 147–149

    brassiness, 148

    highlighting, 147–148

Bubble baths, products, 104–105

    professional selection, 105

C

Calluses. *See* Feet

Camouflage techniques, 64

Cassia betaglycan, usage, 190

Cellulite

    at-home treatment, 101

    solutions, 100

    strategies, 99–101

    treatment, 100–101

    water, impact, 101

Chan, Nelson, xii

Chaste tree, usage, 190

Chest

    anti-aging products, application, 7

    treatment, 7

Chirally correct, definition, 202

Choi, Jin Soon, xii, 165–166

Cholic acid, usage, 197

Chronic dryness, 99

G

Gadberry, Rebecca James, xiii, 2, 16, 107
Gardner, Diane, xiii, 35, 68, 83, 120, 146
Genestein, definition, 202
Giella, xiii, 1, 15, 36, 53, 67, 82, 107, 165
    color chart, 61–62
    color classifications, 60–61
Glick, Hara, xiii, 36, 120
Glossary, 201–204
Glycolic acid, 26
    peel, definition, 202
Grapeseed extracts, 30
Gray hair, 149–150
    disguise, 149
    guidance, 150
    shades, 149
Green, Meredith, xiii, 95
Green vegetables/algae/fruit, consumption, 121
Groomers, products (professional selection), 143–144
Gross, Dennis, xiv, 2, 16, 107

H

Hadley, Skyy, xiv, 166
    secrets. *See* Manicures
Hair. *See* Brunette hair; Curly hair; Fine hair; Frizzy hair; Gray hair; Thick hair
    blow-drying, 133–134
    brushes, usage, 132
    care, 119–122
    damage, prevention, 146
    drying time, 123–124
    dryness, cessation, 130
    green tint, 153–154
    herbs, usage, 147

highlighting, advice, 152–153
highlights, selection, 152–153
ionic treatments, 132
length, 154–155
    color, interaction, 154–155
    errors, 123
mistakes, 122–124
negative charge (ions), 131
pigments, 149
products, principles, 129–131
rinse, 121–122
salon, strategies, 159–162
secrets, 138–139
style
    mistakes, 123
    speed, 126
success, 129–130
tools/techniques, 131–132
trim, schedule/frequency, 124
wooden combs, usage, 132
youthfulness, 127
Hair color. *See* Home hair color
    care, 159
    communication, 157–158
    comprehension, 156
    consultation, 145–147, 157
    contrast, 151
    darkness, problems, 151
    definition, 156
    errors, 150–151
    problems, 122–123
    products, professional selection, 163
    technique, 155–157
        selection, 155–156
    well water, impact, 156
Hair styling, 125–126, 128–129
    errors, 123

knowledge, 8

quality, 7–8

Nd:Yag laser, definition, 203

Neck

anti-aging products, application, 7

care, 7

treatment, 7

Neti pot, definition, 203

Neutral lipstick, usage, 86

Neutrals, usage, 38

Niacinamide, usage, 198

Nice, Angela, xv, 96, 108

Nighttime skin care, 5

No-chip nails, 176–177

Noodleman, Rick, xv, 108

Nose, contours, 40

O

Octyl methoxycinnamate (Parsol MCX), definition, 203

Oily skin, dusting, 47

Olive skin, foundation shade, 44

Ophals, Gabrielle, xv, 16, 95

Oribe, xvi

Ornstein, Michelle, xvi, 83

O'Rourke, Michael, xvi, 119, 146

Ouidad, xvi, 120, 146

Overtweezing, 70

P

Parabens, definition, 203

Paraffin, usage, 167

Parsol 1789. *See* Avobenzone

Parsol MCX. *See* Octyl methoxycinnamate

Pearn, Dee, xvi, 165

Pedicures, 165

Peels. *See* Glycolic acid; Home peel; Jessner peel; Trichloro acetic acid peel

explanation, 17

usefulness, 21

Peptides, 28–29

definition, 203

problems, 28

usage, 28–29. *See also* Polypeptides; Skin care

Perdis, Napoleon, xvi, 35, 52

Permanent hair color, 156

Permanent makeup, 55–57

professional, selection, 56

Perms, 136

Photofacial. *See* Intense Pulsed Light

Pimples

prescriptions, 19–20

treatment, 16. *See also* Undergrounder pimples

Pipino, Ric, xvi

Plants

enzymes, usage, 191–192

extracts, problems, 8

Polypeptides, usage, 193–194

Pomades, products (professional selection), 143–144

Ponytails, 131

Pores. *See* Skin

Post-color treatments, products (professional selection), 162–163

Pout, increase, 85

Powder, 46–47

perfecting, 47

products, professional selection, 51

usage, reduction, 47

V

Vaccinium corymbosum L. *See* Blueberry

Vaccinium macrocarpon. *See* Cranberry

Vanegas, Jimmy, xviii, 120

Vartoughian, Jessica, xviii, 165

    advice. *See* Manicures

Vegetables, enzymes (usage), 191–192

Velcro rollers, usage, 131

ViÈl, Louis, xviii, 145

Vitamin A (Retinol)

    definition, 203

    usage, 194, 198

Vitamin B, usage, 197

Vitamin C, 22

    necessity, 27

Vitamin D, absorption, 109

Vitamin K, definition, 204

W

Warm colors, 59

Washcloths, usage, 10

Waxes, products (professional selection),
    143–144

White bumps. *See* Milia

White spots, warning, 24

Wings, avoidance, 96

Witch hazel *(Hamamelis virginiana),* usage, 199

Worthington, Charles, xviii, 120

Wright, Hollis, xviii–xix, 54

Wu, Jessica, xix, 1, 15, 96, 108

Z

Zeolite, usage, 199

Zinc oxide, definition, 204

Zomnir, Wende, xix, 16, 36, 67, 83, 95, 166

About the Author

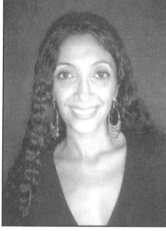

Nada Guirgis Manley is a recognized fashion and beauty writer with over 1,000 magazine articles to her credit. She is also a former beauty editor with more than a dozen years of experience. She has made numerous television appearances as a fashion and beauty expert on FOXNews and E! Entertainment Television. Currently based in central Florida, she is a fashion columnist for the *Daytona Beach News-Journal* and a freelance writer. *Secrets of the Beauty Insiders* is the culmination of her lifelong obsession with beauty. Log on to www.nadamanley.com for more beauty tips, product picks, and upcoming appearances.